THE DANCING HEALERS

A Doctor's Journey of Healing with Native Americans

Carl A. Hammerschlag, M.D.

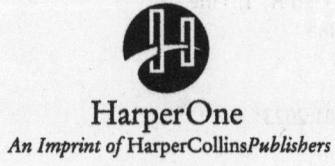

HarperOne
An Imprint of HarperCollinsPublishers

HarperOne

HarperCollins books may be purchased for educational, business, or sales
promotional use. For information, please e-mail the Special Markets Department at SPsales@harpercollins.com.

HarperCollins Web site: http://www.harpercollins.com

HarperCollins®, 🐟®, and HarperOne™ are trademarks of HarperCollins
Publishers.

FIRST HARPERCOLLINS PAPERBACK EDITION PUBLISHED IN 1989

Library of Congress Cataloging-in-Publication Data
    Hammerschlag, Carl A.
      The dancing healers : a doctor's journey of healing with native
    Americans / Carl A. Hammerschlag.
      ISBN 978–0–06–250395–4
      1. Indians of North America—Southwest, New—Medicine.
    2. Hammerschlag, Carl A. I. Title
    E78.S7H23   1988
    615.8'51–dc19   87–45704

            HB 02.01.2023

CONTENTS

PREFACE

Milton Erickson, that master hypnotherapist, understood that to begin a story by saying "Remember when" was already to begin to place the audience into an altered state of consciousness—the very act of remembering is a kind of trance in itself. Erickson also knew that when you tell a story, you are speaking directly to the unconscious, the very essence of the listener.

My twenty years in Indian country have shown me the great, universal power inherent in the stories we have told each other in all cultures throughout all of time. There are heroes; there are monsters. People die; they are reborn. And there are miracles.

When we see this universal connection among all who have walked the earth, it becomes clear that all history is the history of our own time. All stories speak to each of us. Understanding this connection is crucial if we're to be able to live together and to live with ourselves. We must learn to feel how other people connect to one another and to the universe.

No one makes it alone. We must all be connected to something other than ourselves—to others on our walk and to something outside all of us. At the same time, in this everlasting now, each of us is unique. We each have our own truth and our own power, and that is what we must follow.

These are the stories I have lived. They tell of how I began to learn to become a healer rather than a doctor. They tell of how I came to understand that the power to heal comes from hearing your own music and dancing your own dance.

ACKNOWLEDGMENTS

It was the old Indian men who told me that I should tell the stories. It has not been easy. For eight years I have picked the manuscript up and put it down.

Would my motives be suspect? Would I be ridiculed? Would the visibility compromise my credibility?

Enough already. Listen to the stories. They are not mine. I just heard them.

They are all true. I have changed some names and places to protect the anonymity of those who chose to remain unnamed. The words are mine, in the best way I know how to write them. If the stories do not move you, it is because I could not write them as well as I learned them.

I have never seen or walked the path alone. The book is for my family, friends, teachers, patients, and students who have walked with me. It is with love for my wife and children who made the painful and enlightening journey near, if not always by, my side.

It is with thanks to Brad Steiger, Phyllis Steckler, Carol Sowell, Tom Grady, and Ann Moru, who felt my heart and showed me how to share it better. To Dennis Numkena, visionary artist, whose cover design illuminates the Hopi symbols of the healing dance.

And it is for these mentors, their light still shines;

Santiago Rosetta 1893–1975
Arno Hammerschlag 1905–1977
Herbert Talaheftewa 1903–1979
Bill Dalton 1897–1981

Erich Fromm 1900–1980
Milton Erickson 1901–1980
Brave Buffalo (Devere Eastman) 1930–1987

Mi takuye oyacin
To all my relations
C.A.H.

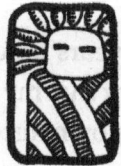 **SANTIAGO'S DANCE**

In 1965, after I had completed my medical internship at the Public Health Service Hospital in Seattle, Washington, I entered the Indian Health Service. It made more sense to me than going to Vietnam, a real possibility for someone who was twenty-six years old in that year and a recent graduate from the Upstate Medical Center in Syracuse, New York. Serving with the IHS would fulfill my military obligation. And since no one knows more than someone who has just graduated from medical school, I went to the Indian country of the Southwest to help, to offer healing to the people.

Yet I was also a child. I was terrified of so many things. I had not yet learned that it is all right not to be always sure of everything.

I was a child of my time, an activist in support of the radical causes and beliefs of that day: end the war, help the underdog, listen to the uncorrupted people who live next to the earth. I wanted to work among people I had feelings for, the disenfranchised and the neglected.

Why I chose an Indian reservation in the Southwest rather than the ghettoes of the Eastern cities in which I had grown up was harder to say. The Southwest rang with a certain mystery; I had a romantic vision of a unique culture. I didn't know then why the Southwest drew me, but I had a sense there was something there to be learned.

And indeed, after more than twenty years among the native people of the Southwest, I now know that my further education, my unfinished business with my own history and my own demons, the things I needed to know to be able to help myself and others—those were the real reasons I came to this beautiful, mysterious country.

During my education at the City College of New York and the State University of New York Medical School, my plan was to be a "real doctor," a family practitioner. I would hang a shingle someplace and let people pay me in chickens and pigs. I thought I could bring healing to plain people who would gratefully welcome my expertness. I was ready to save the world—people needed me. Most of us go into medicine to try to "do it" for somebody.

I didn't know I was going to the Southwest to be healed myself.

The IHS sent me to Sante Fe, New Mexico, as a General Medical Officer assigned to the Pueblo tribes along the Rio Grande. The very name rang with magic! The Rio Grande. How exotic.

I came with a wife and two small daughters. Elaine and I had met when I was nineteen and a premedical student; she was a nurse. It was the familiar doctor-nurse pairing: young nurse marries young med student and helps put him through school. We survived the stresses of the process and managed to transform the struggle into a growing family.

I was a big-city boy from the concrete canyons of the East who thought you needed to be immunized against yellow fever if you were foolhardy enough to cross the George Washington Bridge. I knew nothing of the Pueblo tribes. I knew Indians only from Hollywood's shallow presentations. And in those sagas I had always cheered for the Indians against the cowboys, because of my sympathy for the apparent underdog in any situation.

But Santa Fe immediately began chipping away at my brand new M.D. bravado. It was the smallest town Elaine and I had ever seen, and I found that many of those I had come to help hated me simply because I was a white man. As a child of the Jewish nightmares of World War II, I could certainly identify with the Indians' terrible sense of disenfranchisement, but I could not relate to being hated simply for being white.

I worked in the Santa Fe Indian Hospital under direction of an old doc who had been there for many years. The hospital was a collection of huge wards. You could go from one bed to the next just by moving the "chart cart" six inches down.

The pace was killing. I worked seven days a week. Another young doctor and I were on call every other night and every other weekend. Lunch got eaten while I moved from one room to another. I had expected to work long and hard, but I didn't expect to be seeing one hundred people a day, to have no time to think and no energy for my family. It didn't take me long to realize I wasn't up to the rigors of a life as a general practitioner in that kind of setting.

The conditions we saw were distressing and we functioned in a constant state of emergency. Members of the Pueblo tribes came to us with every kind of ailment—gastric ulcers, tuberculosis, heart attacks, cancers. The rate of infant mortality was high and it wasn't unusual to see children with 5-to-10-percent dehydration, the result of severe diarrhea. These children were so shriveled we had to shave their scalps to find veins where we could inject the intravenous fluid needed to restore health.

Despite these conditions, the Pueblos were reluctant to come to the hospital to see doctors. For them an illness would either get better or it wouldn't and a hospital was a place you went to die.

What we saw as their passivity frustrated us. What we didn't know was that there was another system, another way of dealing with living and dying, suffering and healing, that we knew nothing of. We young smart docs thought we could do more than we really could and knew more than we did.

Since ours was the only medical service and we were the only doctors on the reservation, two days a week I went out into the villages. The Indian Health Service had only started in 1955. Before that, the Bureau of Indian Affairs (BIA) in the Department of the Interior ran such hospitals as there were. And during World War II, Indian facilities were last on the list to receive supplies and personnel. I was unprepared for the results of this long-time neglect.

I saw a rare liver disease in a previously healthy twenty-year-old woman who delivered a quite jaundiced, stillborn child and then died herself within twenty-four hours. It transpired so quickly that I felt I never knew what happened.

I had a patient whose heart valves were being nibbled away by bacteria that had invaded his blood after he had cut himself while skinning a rabbit. In spite of vigorous treatment, I watched him die from blood poisoning in six weeks.

I lost a thirty-year-old chronic alcoholic in delerium tremens. He drowned in his own secretions, an unlikely complication of that disease I had been taught.

There was dying all around me, for which I was not well prepared. It made me worry about my competence and my training. Some people afflicted with a disease got well, while others who suffered from the same malady died from it. Certain men and women who were exposed to a disease never got it at all.

Many of the women delivered their babies squatting on sheepskins so that the first thing the child would touch was the Earth, the mother of us all. They refused to get on the table and give birth on their backs. When they would agree to climb onto the table to deliver the afterbirth, I had to accept this as a reasonable compromise.

Some of what I had learned in medical school seemed to have left my memory completely. One woman who hadn't seen a doctor during her pregnancy delivered an infant daughter, whom I carried to the bassinet for the standard cleansing procedures. As I was cleaning the baby, the nurse called me back to the mother. From the vaginal opening a tiny leg protruded. I ran back to the bassinet: my first thought was that I had delivered the baby but had somehow left one leg behind! The nurse graciously brought the young doctor back to reality by gently advising him that she thought the twin was ready to deliver.

I was still learning so many things, while all around me people were still dying, and as a doctor I took every death personally. Those of us in the medical profession are generally unprepared to deal with death. We view it as some obscene shortcoming in our healing skills. This kind of professional narcissism makes it very hard to heal others. When we professionals think that we are the only ones doing the healing, we are setting ourselves up for pain and disillusionment.

I had not yet perceived the connections of spirit on the part of both patient and doctor that are involved in the total healing process. Neither could I imagine that a person could determine or know the time of his or her death. Then I met Vincente.

Vincente, a traditionalist Indian from Santo Domingo Pueblo, was in his early forties. He complained of soreness in his gut and the loss of considerable weight over the previous five months. Tests revealed that he harbored a malignant stomach tumor. We opened him up and found the tumor everywhere. There was nothing we could do.

Afterward, the incision site never healed properly, and necrotic debris continually oozed out of his belly. I tried to describe what he had and tell him about his odds, but there was no word for cancer in the Pueblos' Keres language, and I was afraid he wouldn't understand the terms in English. I said something about a kind of fire that was spreading out of control and told him that medicine, like water, did not always extinguish the flame.

Almost as if he were turning the subject away from his own mortality, he asked me how far away August 4 was. He was smiling. I thought I must be doing something wrong because Vincente didn't respond to the news of his imminent death the way I would. Instead of denying that he was dying or demanding that I do something about it, he was calmly inquiring about the most important feast day of his village.

I regretted having to say that the event was still two months away since I knew he would be dead before then. Far from the disconsolate response I had feared, he told me without hesitation that he would go home for that feast day. I said, "Fine, Vincente. I'll take you back to Santo Domingo for the ceremony," thinking with all medical certainty that he would never see that day.

But on August 4, Vincente was still alive. I drove him the thirty-five miles from the hospital to Santo Domingo in my station wagon so that he could lie down in the back. I brought dressing changes and painkilling medications with me so that I might tend to him professionally. I helped him into his home, a hot adobe house where his wife and children, other relatives, and friends came in to speak quietly with him. While he visited with these people, my family and I watched the ceremonial dances.

Here was the exotic Southwest I had envisioned. It was like walking out of the subway in New York into a living exhibit from the Museum of Natural History. The colorful clothing, the traditional dances, the tiered adobe houses with ladders propped outside were indeed as romantic as I had imagined.

But it was hard to appreciate the brilliance and grandeur of the Pueblo culture because of the overwhelming poverty of these communities. A few concrete block homes were scattered through the villages, but most were of adobe, and many had crumbling walls and corners. Families lived in one or two small rooms, and few houses had plumbing or electricity, even in the 1960s. Some of the homes had dirt floors, others wooden planks. Families carried and stored their water in fifty-gallon cans. Battery-powered radios, sewing machines, and other appliances sat outside the houses, and much of the living seemed to be a sharing of the communal outdoor spaces.

I would learn, as I lived in New Mexico, that the Pueblo culture differed in many ways from mainstream America — and not just in the absence of conveniences and consumer goods. Young Indians frequently left the pueblos and moved to the cities for school or for jobs; some established families and mortgages in the suburbs of Santa Fe or Albuquerque. Over the years, they would return to attend traditional ceremonies in their pueblos, to recharge themselves by reconnecting with their spiritual roots. As a Pueblo Indian grew older, he or she was expected to take a greater part in the rituals of the community. Parents knew that most of their sons and daughters would be drawn back there eventually by ties of many centuries. Eventually many would come back for good.

On the day I took Vincente to Santo Domingo, I saw people go into his home carrying branches and other objects that I didn't pay much attention to. Later I learned that these people were the priests of his tribe, who sprinkled corn pollen on him, brushed him with spruce branches, and blessed him with ceremonial objects.

Although Vincente was in obvious pain throughout the entire day, he never once asked for a painkilling shot. When it was time to leave, he climbed into the back of my station wagon. He did not say a great deal to his family, but he touched each one of them and waved farewell as we left. I was glad that he'd had a chance to say goodbye in a way that had meaning for him.

Back in his hospital bed that evening, Vincente announced that he was now ready to die. I downplayed his announcement, reminding him what a good day he had experienced. I told him I would see him in the morning. He said, "No. I am going to die."

In the morning I went into Vincente's room. The bed was empty. He had died during the night.

I was unprepared for an experience like this. I had been through medical school, and I knew when people were going to live and die. But this guy knew more about his own life and death than I did. He had handled the whole thing with calm dignity and certainty. That didn't make sense, and I couldn't shake the feeling of bewilderment.

I said to Bob McCormick, my colleague, "You're not going to believe this," and told him Vincente's story. He too found it astonishing, but he didn't seem as baffled as I. I think now it's because Bob was a religious man who was active in his church; he was better prepared to accept the mysterious with faith.

But Vincente's experience made an impression on me. I had a glimmer of a sense that there was something there for me to learn, but I still had no idea what that might be.

Now I know much more about the importance of ritual, the lesson I had begun to learn after watching Vincente orchestrate his farewells and his death in the way he needed to do. Ritual allows us to attach ourselves to the sacred. Sacraments permit us to see and to feel the holy. Corn pollen, sweet grass, incense, rosaries, prayer shawls—they all help us to separate the sacred from the profane or the ordinary. All these physical attachments help us to get in touch with the nontangible aspects of our spirit.

I was beginning to be ready to learn that the spirit plays as big a role in our wellness and sickness as the mind and the body do. I was, by now, becoming quite ripe for Santiago Rosetta.

Santiago, also from Santo Domingo, had been admitted to the Sante Fe Indian Hospital with congestive heart failure.

I didn't know that he was a Pueblo priest and clan chief. I only saw an old man in his seventies lying in a hospital bed with oxygen tubes in his nostrils.

Suddenly there was this beautiful smile, and he asked me, "Where did you learn to heal?"

Although I assumed my academic credentials would mean little to the old man, I responded almost by rote, rattling off my medical education, internship, and certification.

Again the beatific smile and another question: "Do you know how to *dance*?"

Somehow touched by whimsy at the old man's query, I answered that, sure, I liked to dance; and I shuffled a little at his bedside. Santiago chuckled, got out of bed, and, short of breath, began to show me his dance.

"You must be able to dance if you are to heal people," he said.

"And will you teach me your steps?" I asked, indulging the aging priest.

Santiago nodded. "Yes, I can teach you my steps, but you will have to hear your own music."

I was twenty-six years old, just out of medical school, filled with great certainties—however sorely they might be wearing away under the steady corrosiveness of pain and death. To me, at that moment in my spiritual evolution, Santiago sounded like another mystical holy man slightly removed from the realities I had to deal with. But a seed had been planted, a friendship had begun, and I later visited him many times in his home. The seeds that Santiago planted within my psyche would not sprout until I returned East.

In 1967 we left New Mexico so that I might go to Yale and study psychiatry. I had learned in Santa Fe that I wasn't willing to make a career of seeing patients seven days a week and every other night with no time to think or give patients the kind of attention I wanted to. I knew that the mind had much to do with the body's health and I was intrigued by that mystery. I have since learned that the mind will always have a mind of its own; we'll never understand it. But then I wanted to understand all that I could about the mind. Psychiatry held forth the promise of theory and explanation for the internal and eternal mysteries.

But at Yale, I encountered obstinacy as well as mystery. Several experiences showed me that I didn't belong in an urban academic setting. When I applied for a grant from Aid to Dependent Children to supplement the $4,400 a year I earned as a first-year resident, the psychiatry department was upset that the Yale salary structure had been made a matter of public display. August personages interpreted my action as a difficulty with authority that must stem from some unresolved business with my father.

Such psychiatric interpretations are designed to blunt the passion of any action, and I eventually learned not to make them. In psychiatric training, I also learned how to make and present diagnoses and, more important, when to talk and when to keep quiet. I studied the literature, the analysts, the ego-psychologists, the behaviorists, the existentialists, the geneticists, the anatomists, and the biochemists. The more I pondered the theories, the more illusory seemed the ultimate answers about the mind and body that I had hoped to find.

For a time I worked in the new facilities of the Connecticut Mental Health Center, which was situated in the "Hill" area on the fringe of New Haven's black ghetto. This was at the height of black militancy. The Bobby Seale trial had taken place in New Haven, and race riots had erupted in major cities every summer. Black leaders and groups were emerging throughout the country, and part of blacks' growing pride and self-assertion involved a strong distrust or even hatred of whites.

I was dismayed that few of my black patients stayed in treatment for any significant period of time and troubled that they saw me as an enemy. I realized they interpreted my silence during therapy as part of a power game to make them talk first. If I were going to help these people at all, I would have to do it another way.

In my search for an effective solution to the problem, I discovered community psychiatry. This technique said to me, "Get out there and use the whole system to effect change. Address the job, the boss, the school, the family, the street—use everything!" So I conducted an "after-care" clinic on Congress Avenue for people who had been discharged following a hospital stay—I conducted it in bars, on street corners, and especially in barbershops. People talked a lot easier out there too.

Nothing functions by itself, I now realized. Everything is interrelated—body, mind, and spirit. Family, community, country. Job, education, heritage, home. History, culture, religious beliefs, principles. How we put all these together in our lives makes up the unique individuals we are. My role as a therapist was to help people discover their own uniqueness in credible, healthy ways and to find what will sustain them and connect them to the larger reality of human and spiritual experience.

The New Haven race riots erupted four months after my arrival at the Mental Health Center. The center was designated an evacuation center for all the potential "crazies" who might develop as a result of this social confrontation. Interestingly, we had no psychiatric emergencies on those nights. As a matter of fact, there were actually fewer problems than usual.

Perhaps when disaster is imminent, people pull themselves together. Even the so-called crazies get it together. It is as if everybody understands that no one can tolerate madness at such explosive times.

My mentors in the psychiatry department were not pleased when I got arrested for participating in a sit-in at an abandoned city-owned building that community residents wanted to use as a drug detoxification facility—at that time there was no such facility in the city. The department once again interpreted my involvement as another manifestation of my innate problem with authority. I saw my support of the community's expression of its needs as a true demonstration of what community psychiatry was all about.

These and other experiences at Yale showed me that making a difference to people happens in the doing, not in talking about it. The seed of Santiago's wisdom had begun to sprout. He had tried to teach me that if you are going to dance, you have to move. You can't watch the dance; you can't listen to it or look at it. You have to do it to know it.

Yale was an exciting place with opportunities for taking a stand on social issues, but it wasn't the place for me. I wanted to return to the Southwest. There I could practice community psychiatry with respect for and involvement in the community's way of life.

Yet another reason for my desire to return to Indian country was that I had come to identify strongly with the Indians' struggle. I had come to see the Jewish experience as a recapitulation of the Indian experience. You're living peacefully in your home and someone comes and says, "Get off your land and give it to us or we'll kill you!" Indians were survivors, just as my parents had been. They had seen the handwriting on the wall in 1936 and left Germany for America. Their family members who survived were scattered over four continents.

Leaving their home was a wrenching experience for my relatives. My grandfather had won the German Cross in World War I. When I visited him in Israel in 1950, he showed it to me. He still believed that the Germany that had existed before Hitler was a different Germany, a different experience. He was able to distinguish Germany and the German people from the Nazis, something I'd never managed.

I grew up terrified of Germans and, at the same time, angry at Jews and at my own Jewishness. How could all those people have been so weak and intimidated that they would just walk into the ovens? Did this mean that Jews were by their very nature weak and ineffectual people? I used to wonder what I would have done if the Nazis had lined me up for extermination. Would I have resisted? Would I have run? Was I, too, weak?

As a boy, I would squeeze my fingernails with pliers just to see how much pain I could stand before I screamed. I wanted to make myself tough and show my contempt for pain; I also wanted to hide from my fear. Yet I knew that my self-inflicted ordeals really did not matter. Whatever pain or suffering I could endure would never compare to what the victims of Nazi brutality had seen and suffered.

I became preoccupied with fears of anti-Semitism. Whenever I heard people speaking German, I would feel icy claws at my stomach. In elevators or on subways, I would eavesdrop on conversations to see if I could catch anyone making anti-Semitic comments.

None of my family ever openly discussed the concentration camp survivors. That awful time was never mentioned. Whatever had happened was too horrible to speak of ever again. I lived with the horrors and fears and guilt in my imagination.

I struggled through my adolescence complaining as little as possible. I never shared my feelings about pain, the cold, or sadness. When things got really lousy, I got through it by figuring that perhaps now I knew a small portion of the pain of other Jews. Feeling good always made me guilty for not having experienced enough sorrow.

From my efforts to define my identity as a Jew, my growing identification with Indians, and my experiences at the Connecticut Mental Health Center, I found a more certain place for myself as a doctor who could make a difference in a community. Respect for other people's experience and culture was essential before I could offer them anything from my knowledge or experience.

How different the entire history of civilization would have been if the conquerors had only viewed the conquered as having knowledge and experience to be shared. Instead victors assume the conquered have nothing to tell them because they lost, which only reinforces the belief that there is only one viewpoint, one perspective on the way—the way to truth, to knowledge, to life.

We now look to science to provide us with the answers to the Great Questions. But the answers to questions about meaning usually lie within ourselves. If we are comfortable only with answers that can be proven, we'll never really get comfortable. Science is not something to worship. We worship to acknowledge and revere the things we *don't* understand.

Interestingly, it's the physicists, like the priests and visionaries, who accept this "Uncertainty Principle." Nuclear and particle physics yield this new conviction that there are some things you can't predict. Not only does God play dice with the universe, sometimes he rolls them where you can't find them. The search for truth represents a longing, not a destination.

I have come to see clearly that those men and women who survive crises are those who have maintained a special connection to the way. They have walked their own walk with eyes open to the people and the truths around them, without discounting the walks of others. They have developed a special sense of who they are. They have supplemented the knowledge of science with a faith in the mysterious. The lesson they have imparted to me is unquestionably this: if you are going to greet the world as an equal, your feet have to be planted firmly in some unique, prideful recognition of Self. You must learn in a good way that what you are is okay. Then you can know that others are just fine too.

Our civilization has encouraged us to be independent, self-steering, goal-directed. Be your own person. Do your own thing. But sometimes we feel weak. Sometimes we feel human. At those times, we need to know that we are connected to those who came before and to those who will come after us.

This book is about medicine men and women who have helped me to learn. It is about mystery. It is about how psychiatric thinking is culture-bound. It is about the fact that neither science nor psychology has thus far provided us with a cohesive picture of the ways of human experience.

This book describes the inseparability between curing and the sense of the mystical. Healing is a powerful, culturally endorsed ritual. There is no doubt that if you trust the practitioner and if you share the same cultural myths, healing is better achieved. In the final analysis, however, I must admit that the crisis of modern life are no better alleviated by psychiatrists than by visionaries, for both attempt to provide explanations for questions that have no simple answers.

Young Indian people are coming back to reservations and communities of their forebears. They are learning their languages, their songs, their traditions. They are learning how to get connected with who they are historically and spiritually. All of us need to do the same in a way that works; we need to come back to our own truths.

I want this book to enable people to walk their own walk, wherever and whatever it may be. I do not want people to rush to the reservations to walk the Indians' walk. And I most definitely do not want them to pound on my door and insist upon walking my walk. I want each individual to seek his or her own way and to discover a personal truth.

And now the stories I learned in Indian country. I can only share these stories with you. You must set them to your own music.

Chapter 1

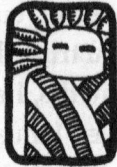 **BASIL**

I came back to the Indian Health Service in 1970 as a civil servant, not as the commissioned officer in the U.S. Public Health Service I had been in Santa Fe.

I remained in Phoenix as Chief of Psychiatry for more than fifteen years. As someone who always had trouble with the rules and the rulers, I cannot really believe it myself. But the Indian Health Service was tolerant of me and supportive of a community-based, preventative mental health program. During my first year in Phoenix, I spent half my time at an Indian boarding school and half at the Indian Medical Center, creating a community-based program that I thought would work.

Traditionally, psychiatry has been defined as a direct service—the doctor sees individuals face to face, makes a diagnosis, prescribes treatment, and follows the patient's progress. As the only psychiatrist to cover not only the reservations spread out through Arizona, but also the Phoenix urban area, I knew there was no way I could see everyone I might be able to treat individually—and the culture itself didn't particularly fit this approach.

I decided I would teach people to help themselves. I said: "This is what I know and if you'd like to know what I know, I'd be willing to teach you. But I also want to learn what you know." So I developed a system of bringing my services to the urban and reservation communities. I got a pilot's license and flew to a different reservation once a week. I taught groups of community health workers, nurses, doctors (and their spouses), Head Start teachers, tribal jailers and inmates, and the participants in alcoholism programs. And in the process, I learned about the history, the beliefs, the lives of people in those communities.

This way I've seen far more people than I could ever have seen one on one. And I've done my job as an equal participant. I expected to learn as much as I taught; I knew these people had much to teach me. And learning from them meant gradually finding out how many things—not just about health or psychiatry—I thought I knew but didn't.

The Indian boarding school in Phoenix, where I worked half-time during my first year in Phoenix, was largely populated by youngsters sent there from their reservations for some "problem." Either they didn't get along in the public schools or their parents couldn't afford to keep them at home. For a time, our government had forced all Indian children to live in boarding schools away from home and tribal roots in an effort to make Anglo-Americans out of them. Now there are schools on most reservations, so the off-reservation boarding schools are a last resort for children or families with problems.

When I returned to the Southwest, I believed that the opportunity to work with young people would give me with the greatest opportunity to effect change. But this school, with its troubled students, proved to be too tough a place to accomplish very much. Little true learning went on because teachers and students spent most of their time struggling with each other for control of the classroom.

During my year there, I conducted a "training group" for high-school juniors and seniors. The class was billed as a "participatory learning experience," and each student received academic credit from the Social Studies Department. Fifteen students enrolled in this class, an experimental course entitled "Understanding Human Behavior."

At this time the spirit of the black revolution had just begun to reach the young Indians, and on the first day the room was full of anger. Among the pupils was Basil, who sported a headband and long braids. He was sixteen, and he didn't like me at all. It was not that Basil distrusted me; he really did not like *me*.

His opening comment to the group was that I was just another white man who had come to "lay down some more bullshit." If I had hoped to raise the consciousness of these students and get them to react, I had misunderstood the process.

Basil was not the subservient, unemotional, dependent, powerless Indian I had expected to meet. He was challenging, hostile, competitive, and the rest of the class clearly approved of what he was saying and doing to the teacher. I pulled my chair into the middle of the circle and told the students that I felt surrounded, as if I were their enemy. I complained that I did not like such treatment.

"I don't see myself as just another white man," I told them. "As a matter of fact, I had never seen myself as a white man until I came to the Southwest. I have always been a Jewish man."

I explained that I had my own history quite separate and distinct from that of any other white person they knew, and I challenged them to wait to make up their own minds about me when they knew me better.

"Just another honky scam," Basil snorted to the class. "Now they're sending some headshrinker to try to brainwash us."

"Basil," I laughed, teasing him, "you're probably Sanforized, so you're shrinkproof."

That was how the class began, and I learned something very important. If you are going to survive in Indian country, you have to learn how to deal with anger. It is laudable for teachers to tell Indian children about the past glories and noble traditions of the red man, but the truth is that what Indian children have seen for the past one hundred years of their history is not glory and greatness, but despair and disenfranchisement.

And now there was Basil hating me simply because I was white. He knew nothing of my pains, hopes, dreams, and aspirations. My being white was enough to make me eligible for his total prejudice.

Feeling Basil's uncensored anger that day was a jarring experience for me, and one of its effects was to force me to confront my own ugly racism that said all Germans were Nazis and no Christian could be trusted. Every time you actually think that you've got it together, something occurs to remind you not to take yourself so seriously. I was a welltrained, alledgedly ecumenical, nonjudgmental psychiatrist who, in dealing with someone else's prejudice, was forced once again to confront his own.

As a kid, my determining criterion for friendship was whether you would hide me in your attic if the Nazis ever came after me. That was my price for intimacy, my "Anne Frank" method of evaluating loyalty. It turned out to be a good way not to get too close to anyone. I think Jews often share a certain pride about suffering that we really don't want to give up. It's like a badge of honor: "We've suffered more than you."

I had basically settled the Christian business quite some time ago, forgiven them as a whole, and been able to become intimate friends with non-Jews. Except for Germans. Germans were always another story. Whenever I heard people speaking German, I would still quietly listen to their conversation, waiting for some anti-Semitic slur. Basil and the class of Indian students forced me to confront my own hatreds, and I have continued to struggle with those feelings ever since.

In 1983 at a tropical resort I was watching the sun set while listening to a classical music concert by the shore and reading Yaffa Eliach's *Hasidic Tales of the Holocaust*. This book, the first compilation of Hasidic stories in generations, touched me profoundly on several levels of my being through tales that once again described the reality of the horrors my family had lived through but also through stories of kindness, friendship, even laughter.

Next to me, reclining in another lounge chair, was a young woman who was also listening to the concert and watching the sun set. At the end of the performance, she leaned over and in a distinctly German accent asked if I was reading *The Holocaust*. The American mini-series of that name, she explained, had recently been shown on German television.

"No," I said, sitting up straighter (so that I might be better prepared to attack her), "these are Hasidic tales of the Holocaust. They have nothing to do with the television series. By the way," I asked, preparing to pluck an arrow from my quiver of anti-German insults, "what did you think of the television presentation?"

"I was overwhelmed," she replied in a frank and open manner. "It was, of course, all before my time. I knew very little of the period, and I must say that it has been dramatically underrepresented in German school books."

I told her that I spoke German, but rarely to Germans. However, if she were more comfortable I could converse with her in that tongue. Then, with disregard for any kind of social amenity, I told her of my great distrust, even hatred, of all Germans.

She was shocked by my vehemence. She protested that I had never been to Germany, that I had never spoken to young Germans. How could I be so angry toward a people I did not really know?

The image of my days with Basil ten years earlier flashed in my mind, but before I could examine it, I pressed on in my anger and told her a story about my parents' return to Germany in 1960. They had both come from the same small Prussian village, and they had gone back to settle some reparation business. The mayor welcomed them and presented them with flowers. As they wandered the old streets, my parents looked with tears at landmarks and memories.

They stopped at their next-door neighbors' house, and they were astonished to discover that, although quite elderly, the same people still lived there. There were tears and shouts of joy, and these elderly Christians invited my parents inside.

As they walked into the front room, my mother saw a familiar chair sitting in the corner. It was unmistakably her father's rocking chair, abandoned and forgotten in their fearful escape. When the neighbors saw that my mother recognized the chair, they explained that they had taken it from the house because the Nazis would have taken it anyway.

My mother walked out of the house and went back to the railroad station to await the next train. When it pulled out of the village, she dropped the mayor's flowers over the side. She never went back.

When I finished the story, I knew that I had experienced pain and at the same time much joy in telling it. Suffer! Writhe! I thought as I excused myself for dinner.

Just before the next evening's twilight concert, the young woman came up to me and told me that she had cried most of the night. "I cried for your pain," she said softly.

But her words made me flash in anger, so I snapped back at her, "Cry for *your* sins!"

Her firm, quiet reply was not the least bit defensive. "I am not guilty for the sins of my father."

Her words sparked an echo in my mind. It was the same thing I had said to Basil ten years earlier.

When the concert began, I retreated again into my book of Hasidic stories. This time I felt their messages about tenderness, about miracles, about human possibilities in the face of suffering. They were tales not just of horror, but of hope.

But I rejected any positive aspects of the horror stories because I had not wanted to assuage my anger. Like so many men and women, I had been replaying an old script to reexperience old suffering. I would wear it like a faded badge of honor.

When the concert ended, I made the young German woman a gift of my book of Hasidic tales. On the inside cover I inscribed, "Thank you for helping me to continue my work."

The work is never over.

Chapter 2

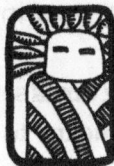 **HERBERT**

Millions of years ago volcanic eruptions from the San Francisco peaks in north-central Arizona covered Hopiland with a hard, dry crust. Rocks eroded by age and water became mesas and canyons, some so deep that they remain dark even in sunlight.

At least one thousand years ago, an ancient farming people who called themselves the Peaceful Ones settled here after a migration that, according to their stories, lasted for thousands of years. Like others who wandered in the desert, the Hopis believed themselves to be a chosen people.

The Great Spirit, Masauwu, the guardian of this, the Fourth World, guided the Hopi to a land where settled humans could exist only by the most delicate of margins, raising nourishment in a dry and difficult land. The Hopi were instructed to stay here, and they established Oraibi and Shungopavi, the oldest continually inhabited villages in North America.

Under the inspiration of Masauwu the Hopi were divided into clans, each with its own legends and rituals that would enable them to maintain balance and harmony in this harsh land. Each generation, it was said, was to perform the rituals and ceremonies in the same manner that the Spiritual Creator had first shown them. Sternly, Masauwu decreed that the Hopi way was not to pass into the hands of others.

The Hopi religion isn't practiced just during times set aside for regular services. Like all religions are meant to do, it involves every aspect of its practitioners' lives. To follow the Hopi way is to live a life of harmony with oneself and with one's surroundings.

Anthropologists cite the Hopi way as the only indigenous belief system to have survived the Anglo-Christian conquest of North America. In the United States, the Hopi religious expression remains the sole surviving taproot of an ancient American spiritual vision.

Over the last century, however, a steadily growing number of Hopis have abandoned their ancient beliefs in favor of the white pattern of economic development. Today, most Hopi are wage earners rather than farmers.

The traditional Hopis complain that working off the reservation makes it difficult to pass on the duties of priesthood in the kiva religious societies. If the next candidate in succession for the priesthood is unavailable for the requisite practice and the exact preparation, when the old priest dies, the ceremony must simply end. And progressive elements within the Hopi have controlled the tribal government since the creation of the elected Hopi Tribal Council under the impetus of the Bureau of Indian Affairs in 1936.

Tribal traditionalists, however, continue to initiate hereditary leaders through the Bear clan. According to the Hopi way, the Creator passed the keys of survival into the hands of the village chiefs, the Kikmongwi, thousands of years ago. To lose the Hopi path here, in the planet's spiritual center, would be to sow the seeds of Earth's destruction.

Herbert Talahaftewa was of the Eagle and Forehead of the Sun clans. As spiritual leader of the two-horned society, he was responsible for the manhood initiation ceremony. I met Herbert shortly after I first came to Arizona. I had heard that he was a highly respected medicine man, a specialist in bones and joints. His services were requested by tribes as far away as the state of Washington.

Herbert was a master of manipulation of the skeleton; he also used poultices, prayers, and the application of hot stones and herbs. He cured many ailments this way, but when a problem did not respond to his methods or he knew he didn't know what to do, he told patients to see the white doctor at the white hospital. He didn't exclude other ways of looking at a problem.

Herbert was also a holy man. He had been initiated into this way by clan predecessors. Nowadays there are schools for medicine men, an idea Herbert scoffed at. To him, the power to heal was a gift. If you received it, then you could practice it and pass it on. You didn't choose to learn it; it found you.

When I was first introduced to Herbert, he was sitting at a loom weaving a ceremonial sash—for among the Hopi it is the men who weave—and wearing a baseball cap bearing with the insignia of the Caterpillar company. He had a twinkle in his eye and a cigarette dangling from a corner of his mouth, and he appeared to be in his sixties. He didn't strike me as particularly holy looking.

Herbert lived in Shungovapi, on Hopi Second Mesa. It's known as a "grandfather village," one of the most traditional

Indian villages on the reservation. Second Mesa is known for its jewelry and weaving and for Herbert's wife, Evangeline, a famous basketmaker. Herbert lived comfortably farming, weaving, and going where he was needed to heal. He lived as a religious leader who was revered in his village.

The introductions were made by a friend, who told Herbert that I was a psychiatrist, a doctor who specialized in the mind. This nugget of information did not appear to impress Herbert in any appreciable way.

When he finally turned to me, he asked, "What do you know about the mind?" His tone was one of amazement, rather than contentiousness. And I was suddenly at a loss for words. In all my training, I had never before been asked that question.

I wanted to appear competent and knowledgeable—wanted him to like me. Should I launch into a lecture about the hypothalamus, the biological determinants of behavior, neuropeptides? Somehow I did not think any of that would impress him. I could not think of a short, incisive answer.

"I guess," I replied after a painful pause, "I really don't know a whole lot about it, I mean, that can be answered briefly . . . in a short time."

Herbert smiled and went back to his weaving. He appeared to be dismissing me with his silence. (In white society, we think something is happening when people are talking. In Indian country, they know something is happening when there is silence.)

I looked around at the walls seeking some kind of solace for my awkwardness. I saw kachina carvings, pictures of children, assorted rattles. I had bungled this opportunity to become acquainted with a respected medicine man.

After what seemed to be a slice of eternity, Herbert turned to me and solemnly pronounced: "If you cannot say what you know about the mind in a short time, then you know nothing of it."

My immediate inner response was anger. This old man had just reduced all my years of education to inconsequence.

"What I know of the mind," Herbert went on, "I can tell you in one word." He paused for a moment. "Mysterious."

Mysterious. The human mind was mysterious. Herbert had looked at the question of what is mind from another perspective, from the aspect of what we don't know. It was an important lesson for me. What I know about it, he was saying, is *I don't know it*.

I wanted to learn what Herbert could teach me. I was open to him, and happily he was willing to talk, then and many times after. I call him my spiritual father. He would not make me a Hopi medicine man but he could teach me some things about the Hopi ways so I could better understand them.

In the years that we worked together after that initial meeting, Herbert often reminded me about what my studies had *not* taught me about the mind. In his opinion, schools, especially those of "higher education," attempted to teach things that were really unfathomable. Indeed, such institutions, by the very presumptuous act of pronouncing themselves "higher," supported the notion that their students could learn higher thoughts than those who had not studied there.

Herbert explained it this way: "We are like long, thin stalks of corn capped with a single gigantic ear. If the 'head' gets too big, the stalk cannot support it. Universities pay attention only to the heads and no attention to the stalks." It is the stalk that carries the spirit to the head.

According to Herbert, we have to learn from the ground up. We must be firmly rooted in the earth, because it is the real teacher. All "heads" need to be solidly connected to their "roots." To learn effectively, both the stalk and the roots must be nurtured.

During this time, in the mid 1970s, I was subjected to a series of debilitating back operations after I had suffered a badly "slipped disc," which had left my leg weak and caused my foot to drop. The surgeries had marked me with serious nerve root scarring and left a ballooning out of the lining of the spinal cord, which kept me from moving easily. I was immobilized with pain, because the drugs I had used to control the pain had stopped being effective. I had begun to prepare for a fourth operation, believing in my heart that the scalpel could cure my chronic pain by correcting the anatomic defect.

This experience of pain and what I would do to deal with it was a major watershed in my life. For the first time I was a cripple, and I wanted to be whole and mobile again. There are always two ways to look at pain: either you've got it, or it's got you. I believed that I was still athletic and strong. If only some skilled surgeon would apply the proper cut, I would be free of pain and normal again.

In retrospect, I know that I never really considered what I was doing to contribute to or intensify my pain. Basically, I was concerned only with keeping my strength up, so that when my back healed I could return to the court as a competitive racquetball player.

A week prior to the scheduled surgery, my secretary called me while I was away at a remote reservation community. She told me that Herbert was in my office and needed to see me. I spoke with him briefly and arranged to meet him in my office the following morning. That morning he asked me if I knew why he was there. I told him I didn't know what he was talking about.

Herbert didn't know why he was there either, but he had had a dream the night before last that had convinced him of his need to see me. Taking the bus to Phoenix was no small commitment for him to make in the middle of the planting season, so I knew that this visit was a true expression of how much the man cared for me.

Herbert continued talking so we could try to understand what had drawn him to visit me. On the day before his dream, he had gone to his fields to look after his first spring planting, only to discover that his seedlings had been destroyed by worms. That night he dreamed that I was standing in a shallow pit in his fields. I was covered by a grey shroud. Maggots were crawling up my legs. My mouth was wide open, but no words were coming out.

Herbert asked me again if I knew why he saw me in the dream. What was happening that would make him aware of me? I told him that I was about to be readmitted to the Mayo Clinic for surgery.

Herbert shook his head in understanding. "You are not to have this surgery. Your head is planted on a decaying stalk, my friend. It is your spirit, not your body, that needs healing."

In his own language, Herbert explained it was time for me to stand up and walk in truth. Pain doesn't go away by telling your mouth not to scream. There are some things you will no longer do, I heard him saying. The pain in your legs is telling you to stop pursuing those old messages. Lifting weights and playing competitive sports are not the only definitions of competence.

I took Herbert to the bus station. He had given me the dream, and now he had to return to the planting. I was moved by Herbert's caring, by the trouble he went to to help me. But I still wasn't ready to let go of my old dreams.

I went to the Mayo Clinic anyway, that sprawling supermarket of modern medicine. I could see in my mind the adhesions that crippled me, and I knew that if they were removed, I would be better. I knew, I believed that I could not get well without surgery.

Doctors repeated the tests. More spinal injections, more corroboration of the spinal sac deformity. I was told that I had a fifty-fifty chance for operative success.

I'm a doctor. I know that nobody goes to elective surgery with those odds. The postoperative complications alone offered the same risks as did the hoped-for cure. I still requested surgery.

A beloved friend had come to be with me. "Shmuck!" he yelled at me. "You go to elective surgery when the odds are ninety-five to five, not fifty-fifty!" He asked the surgeon what would happen without an operation. Would the back continue to deteriorate?

I had never asked that question, because I only wanted to hear that the answer was yes. That way I could fully justify placing myself in the surgeon's hands and having him "do it" to me.

The surgeon explained that my back would wear down faster than normal whether he operated or not. And, when asked if the pain could lessen without surgery, he said that with care and appropriate exercise it could. The surgeon really didn't want to operate, and my friend kept telling me I was crazy. Both of them sounded suspiciously like Herbert.

Still unconvinced but beginning to recognize the evidence, I left the clinic without surgery the next day and went to New York to see a psychiatrist, an expert in bioenergetics, with whom my friend had worked. Lying on a bed, I told the psychiatrist of my anguish, my pain, my crippledness. He imperturbably scratched his nose, and I irritably asked if he was listening to anything I was saying. He admitted that he hadn't heard much.

I wanted to leap off the bed and kill the son of a bitch but I couldn't move. "You insensitive, incompetent fraud," I screamed. "I could strangle you."

He calmly picked up a towel, twisted it, and threw it at me, motioning to me to go ahead. I became enraged. I struggled to my feet and wrapped the towel around his throat and pulled until he gasped. Only then did he push my hands away.

"Well, I'm pleased to see that you can stand," he said calmly.

Not until that moment was I aware that I was pain free! My rage had obliterated the pain. It was the most profound therapeutic intervention I'd ever had. He didn't explain or interpret my problem. He led me to express the rage I didn't know was entangled with my pain.

Symptoms—including pain—are just ways of saying something that, if you could find a way to say straighter, would make the symptoms go away. As a psychiatrist, I knew that. But I didn't know it as a patient. I thought it was something that happened to other people.

I spent the next two weeks recuperating in an upstate New York healing place where I spoke freely about frailty and fear, about Nazis and personal weaknesses. I examined the tyranny of illusions—for example, keeping my pain as another test to prove that I wasn't really afraid. No traditional healer I ever knew had to prove how tough he was.

My back pain sometimes returns, but it's never as severe as it was at that time. I can manage it; I can nurture myself with rest when I begin to feel the symptoms. I can feel it as an old friend tapping me on the back, reminding me to take care of business, to look at my life and where I'm going. Look down and get planted in truth. Listen to what you are saying to yourself.

Herbert had his own personal crisis a short time later.

The progressive leaders of the tribe had endorsed a plan for establishing indoor plumbing in the Hopi villages. They did not believe that the presence of indoor plumbing and hot water took anything away from their being Hopi.

Herbert argued that the sewer lines would disrupt invisible linkages between the kivas and between the kivas and every Hopi home. Kivas are the underground ceremonial chambers where the Kachinas, the supernatural spirits through which humankind and God communicate, live when they visit each summer. All that is sacred in the Hopi tradition is sustained in the kivas. The connections between the kivas and the Hopi had been decreed at the time of the village's creation, Herbert reminded the others. To disrupt them was to separate the heart (the kivas) from these life-sustaining veins that reached into every home on the mesa.

Herbert said that if the connections were broken by this seduction of convenience, it would signal the destruction of the Hopis' special covenant with the Creator. You don't exchange lifelines for sewage disposal. To him, it was that simple.

The village went ahead with the sewer project. So Herbert took another kind of action—he lay down in front of the bulldozer. The construction crew threatened to roll over him, but Herbert wouldn't move. They said they would seek an injunction from Tribal Court and then return. There were no statutory precedents relating to invisible underground connections.

Soon after the encounter, Herbert had a heart attack while in the kiva. He had been fasting and preparing for a ceremony when he simply keeled over. He was over seventy years old. One of the other participants revived Herbert with cardiopulmonary resuscitation. After a brief hospitalization, he was discharged.

Although less active, he still did carpentry work around the house. He was consumed with concern that with white people, Bahaanas, forcing their way into their sacred land, many Hopis would abandon their difficult way. Prophecy had told him that if the Hopi no longer respected their traditions, the land would shrink to nothing.

To Herbert and others, these ancient prophecies were coming true. Fewer young Hopis were passing through the final initiation in which they were given their true Hopi names—not because they didn't want to, but because there were few left who could perform the ceremony properly.

Herbert spent more time alone in the house. He was a traditional chief whose life had been restored in the kiva, and everyone looked at him now with a mixture of awe and fear. He had always been a powerful figure, but his death and rebirth experience had given him a ghostlike quality. Herbert too felt the distance, and we talked about it.

Then one day, as suddenly as it had happened in the kiva, Herbert died from a massive blood clot to his lungs.

I visit his gravesite regularly. It sits below the mesa, and like the others it's covered with sand, stones, and pieces of pottery. The Hopi don't encourage visitors to their cemeteries. When I go to see Herbert, I don't stay long. I tell him I'm feeling better.

In the distance, the silence is broken by the noise of the sewerline machinery.

Chapter 3

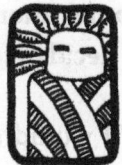 **PROUD MARY**

One day as I was leaving Dilkon, a remote Navajo reservation town just off Arizona Highway 87, I saw a pretty, long-haired young woman hitchhiking. As the father of three daughters, I am very uneasy about female hitchhikers. Too many of them end up violated.

She seemed to be intent upon leaving Dilkon, which is situated halfway between the Hopi Second Mesa villages and the city of Winslow. In the huge expanses of land that make up Arizona's Indian reservations, villages are many miles apart. There is only one major road through this part of this reservation, and the only place it leads is to Winslow, which I had to pass through on my way back to Phoenix. She had to be going my way.

"Hop in," I told her as I pulled my van over.

She accepted my hospitality without a word. Once inside the van, she looked very young, and I felt good that I had stopped for her. Her features were not finely chiseled in the classic Roman way, but she was pretty in a softer, less angular way. She wiped her nose on her sleeve, and I pointed to the box of tissues that I always kept in the van.

"I only want a ride from you," she said sharply. "Nothing else."

Jeez, I save this young woman from a fate worse than death, and in return I get snarls instead of appreciation. After a few more miles of silence, she apparently decided to make herself even clearer.

"If I had a choice," she stated bluntly, "I wouldn't have taken a ride from you or from any white man."

You didn't have to be a psychiatrist to see that she was troubled. I would conveniently serve as the immediate scapegoat—I'd been in Indian country long enough to play that scene patiently.

"The white man destroyed this place of harmony," she continued. "They always took more than they needed." On and on. Not at all a participatory conversation. She was very bright.

When she stopped her invective, I didn't feel as if I had anything to say—or for that matter anything to apologize for. I just nodded so she would know I heard her.

At Winslow, I pulled the van in in front of a cafe. After a few minutes of maintaining a solitary vigil in the van, she joined me inside.

"I agree with some of your ideas," I told her, now that she seemed willing to listen because she wanted to eat. "But I have worked here long enough to know that it isn't only the white people whose values have become distorted. Look at your reservation," I challenged. "It's littered with broken glass, tin cans, garbage. You've lost the path too. Being out of balance, existing in disharmony, is not a disease that favors one color of skin."

It was my turn now, and I was warming to the occasion.

Perhaps she was only quiet because she was eating her hamburger, but I took advantage of the fact that she was chewing on her sandwich and not on me.

"All people are interested in the same things," I waxed on. "We all want a place to sleep, a family, and children to give at least as much to as we ourselves have been given. These basic desires really make us all the same."

The young Navajo's response to my pontification was to belch and walk out of the cafe. I paid the tab, then joined her back in the van. If my conversation was not acceptable, if my skin color was not desirable, at least my wheels were still considered necessary. As we headed out of Winslow, she asked me what I did for a living.

"I am an interpreter of dreams," I replied.

Her response: "Blow it out your ass."

The remainder of the ride went more quickly though the conversation was no warmer. I dropped her off at a convenience market inside the Phoenix city limits and waved goodbye.

Another embittered young Indian, wrapped in anger and confusion.

Some weeks later, a "Mary" left a number with my secretary. I didn't recognize the name, but when I returned the call, the voice at the other end of the line asked me to remember her.

"Remind me."

"I liked the ride down from Dilkon."

Aha! The voice came back to me. So my bright but bitter passenger was named Mary. I truly was surprised to hear from her but delighted that she wished to talk to me about her career plans.

"How about lunch sometime next week?" I offered.

"That would be wonderful," she accepted.

We continued our lunches for two years. Mary told me her story, and I told her mine.

As a child, Mary had sat with her oldest sister night after night waiting for their mother to come home. Mama had grown tired of waiting for Daddy to come home from the tavern, so she joined him and they both drank. Eventually, both would be driven home in the back of some relative's pickup truck. Mary excused her mother: perhaps she really had no choice. With twelve children to support and unable to change her husband's behavior, she gave up too.

It is impossible to talk about Indians without talking about alcoholism. Some theorists say that the 50-to-90-percent rate of alcoholism on the reservations results from a genetic proclivity to metabolize alcohol in a damaging way. I see it differently.

Drinking is another way to suckle nurturance, I told Mary. Nobody makes it alone in the world; we all need something to depend on. If beliefs and traditions don't provide good ways to meet our needs for dependency, we become vulnerable and seek other, more destructive sources of nurture.

Many Indians have been separated from what they believe in by the domination of another culture and by poverty and discrimination. When individuals find little to sustain them in being Indian, the bottle helps them escape the reality.

Once Indians used alcohol as a sacrament in specific rituals, but when a sacrament is misused, it destroys the user. Whether this suicidal process goes slowly or fast, I told Mary, it stems from a simple desire to be heard and an inability to find anyone to listen. If you can discover ways of talking about your feelings more directly to someone you like and believe in, most symptoms disappear—except for the damage done to the body in the meantime.

Mary's father had been found frozen to death in a ditch, another alcoholic death. Her mother continued to drink alone. When Mary was four, she and her siblings were split up, and she was placed in an off-reservation home. This was not an uncommon way for large Indian families to manage when there just wasn't enough money to feed everyone.

Mary's earliest recollections of her new white family included picnics and church. She loved her new life, even though she had readily perceived that she was different from everyone else in her new environment. Church reassured Mary that if she believed, sooner or later she would become "whitesome and delightsome." Mary had convinced herself that as she grew older, her skin would turn paler.

It never happened, and by thirteen she had become a sullen management problem. Mary would get into fights with teachers as well as classmates. She would dare those in authority to do something to her.

In one sense, Mary's trouble stemmed from the ordinary questions of the adolescent in search of an identity: Who am I? What do I really believe in? Mary's queries were complicated by the fact that she was not firmly planted in any unique sense of self. She was unsure of who she was ethnically or where her true home was.

Mary was angry at her white mother for adopting her. She was angry with her Navajo mother for abandoning her. She had completely lost touch with her family on the reservation. As she searched for herself in this conflicting background, her schoolwork deteriorated and she began to steal from her adoptive parents.

When Mary declared that she wanted to go to Indian boarding school, her social worker thought that the Indian identification might be helpful. Her adoptive parents agreed, for she had now exceeded their capacity to deal with her.

At the school, Mary discovered other young Indians who had been sent there from extreme poverty, from alcoholic abuse, from non-English-speaking families, from problems in public schools. They came from a variety of tribes and from diverse backgrounds. What most of them had in common was some problem fitting in where they had been.

Indian boarding schools are frequently understaffed and exhibit a critically low morale. Consequently, the teachers do not teach a lot; the students do not learn a lot; and very little behavior is controlled or constructively modified. Mary had been a scholastic star before her troubled teens had set in motion her downhill slide. In the boarding school she became an academic jewel.

But her identity struggle just became more complicated. The teachers loved her, but Mary did not fit in with the other students. She looked like the rest of them, but she was verbally proficient while most of the others were sullen and silent. Mary could not find happiness in a place where her peers either ignored or ridiculed her.

One day during her first year in boarding school, Mary went shopping in a nearby mall. In a drugstore, she bent down to hold a tin of shoe polish next to her boots to see if the colors matched. The store manager appeared and asked her if she intended to steal the shoe polish. Mary answered unhesitatingly that she was just matching the colors, but he was convinced that she was lying. He next accused her of stealing the items in her shopping bag that she had bought from the department store next door.

Even after the department store personnel verified that Mary had paid for the items, the drugstore manager wasn't satisfied. His clear prejudice wouldn't relent. He told Mary that even if she didn't steal the shoe polish, he knew she was thinking about it. Officiously, he ushered her out the back door, telling her not to come back.

Mary cried with rage, first at him, then at whites. She beat trees, cursed, turned over garbage cans, scrubbed her room to expend some of the seemingly endless rage held in from a lifetime of not belonging.

Then she started a chapter of a militant Indian organization. Her identity was becoming clear—she knew she was Indian. However she was seen by the world, she would flaunt her Indianness, her way. She got buttons, emblems, and bumper stickers. She sent away for posters of American Indian chiefs and sold them at the school.

It doesn't really matter how you get your anger out, only that you get it out. For Mary, anger turned out to be the catalyst to finding the long-needed answer to the question, "Who am I?"

At eighteen, after finishing school, Mary hitchhiked to an Indian commune in California where the people called her "Proud Mary" after the Creedence Clearwater Revival's popular song. At that time, in the mid-seventies, large numbers of young Indians were struggling with what it meant to be Indian. From their political movement, spiritual communities arose, where the young studied the elders' stories, dances, and cosmology. During her time in the commune,

Mary contacted a social worker who helped her locate her biological family.

Mary returned to Dilkon, hitchhiking again. At the town's only store she asked if they knew of her family. In halting English, they pointed out the direction.

Mary walked two miles to a compound comprised of a wooden house, a separate earth and wood hogan, and surrounding corrals. She walked past the chickens, dogs, and bloody sheepskins to approach an old woman sitting in front of the house. This old woman could be her mother. Mary was overwhelmed with that awareness. She didn't know how she would react.

Mary waved at the woman and tried to converse. There was no response, except for a shrug of the shoulders. The old woman understood no English.

Another woman came into the compound with a group of children. Luckily they all spoke English. After a few minutes of conversation, it became clear that this was Mary's sister, together with her nieces and nephews. The two sisters hugged and cried.

In the next hours she learned that her other brothers and sisters had returned home after their first years in foster placement. Only Mary had been adopted.

The family told Mary's mother in Navajo that this stranger was her youngest daughter, the little girl she had given away long ago. But no matter how many ways they told her, the woman didn't remember having another child. The years of alcohol, poverty, and pain had taken their toll on her mind.

What Mary had hoped to get from her mother, a sense of home and belonging, her mother could no longer give. But

Mary could get those things from the rest of her family, who eagerly welcomed her back. Her brothers and sisters wanted to sponsor a welcoming-home ceremony. Mary was overjoyed by the prospect. This was the fulfillment of her search for a place where she belonged.

The ritual of the ceremony helped to heal the rift, the many lost years that Mary had suffered. Now she could begin to know her self, to be whole. By the time I met Mary, she had learned that you can have your feet planted in more than one place and still know who you are.

Navajo medicine men and women use ritual to help restore mental and physical health. They do not reject Western medical or psychological concepts—they only see them as limited. They see the universe as filled with many enormously powerful forces, all of which hold the potential for good and evil. If, for some reason, the balance between good and evil is upset, people get sick. You have to keep in balance if you want to stay healthy.

Mental health is the same way. It can be described as having your head, mouth, and heart in a straight alignment. Mental health happens when what you believe in your heart is the same as what you say with your mouth. You are mentally healthy when what you feel is something you also believe. When the alignment isn't straight, when the mouth doesn't say what the heart feels or when the head knows something the heart doesn't choose to acknowledge, then sooner or later you will get sick.

The traditional Navajo ceremony that Mary's family held to welcome her back helped to restore Mary's balance—and theirs too. This was the way in which they could come together again and Mary could become whole.

The ceremony was held in a hogan. Mary was frightened that she would make mistakes and not be able to repeat exactly the words of the prayers. Her sister helped her learn her part in the ritual.

The medicine man knew every word for the entire ceremony in exactly the right order, each line with its appropriate melody. As he sang, he sprinkled multicolored sands on the ground with movements of his thumb and forefinger, creating what many believe to be the greatest folk art on this continent.

Mary stared at the sand painting in awe. It depicted a Navajo legend about a child who was lost to the tribe, but who returned in another form. The medicine man asked Mary to sit in the middle of the painting. Now she could actually mingle with the heroic figures and absorb their strength.

The medicine man tied feathers and spruce on Mary and placed stone and wooden fetishes, holy objects, on her. He twirled a wooden noisemaker and made a huge roar. Mary felt the breeze from this instrument as if it were blowing her old confused and angry self away.

The medicine man gave her a pipe filled with sweet tobacco. He smoked it; she smoked it; and they blew clouds of tobacco smoke over themselves and toward the sky. For everyone, the atmosphere was charged with feeling.

This was how Mary's odyssey ended. She could like flush toilets, watch television, become well educated, and still be Navajo. She could perceive the world as angry and hostile or as nurturing and sustaining. She had the choice. She could always connect with the things that really mattered. Mary now works among her Navajo people as a health professional.

When we met, Mary was filled with anger at her own exploitation, then anger at white people. She finally gave up the anger. All of what she was served to remind her not to close her eyes to other realities. By hearing all the voices within herself, Mary made a new friend.

Mary kept the parts of herself in alignment by remembering the words sung in her ceremony:

> Happily—may you walk with God—
> Happily—may you walk—
> Happily—may you feel light within—
> Happily—with feeling may you walk—
> Happily—may you walk with God.

All of us need to connect with authentic paths home.

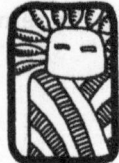

Chapter 4

MILTON AND ERICH

$\mathbf{P}$atty had been referred to me from the hospital's emergency room with "self-inflicted burns." She sat in my office staring at her hands, her straight, shoulder-length hair covering her face like a shroud. She looked about twelve years old but she was nineteen, and four months pregnant. Her husband had brought her to the emergency room after he had found her sticking lighted matches into her navel.

Patty told me that a hummingbird had flown into her bedroom window and had somehow gotten stuck behind the dresser mirror. In trying to escape, the hummingbird had broken its neck. She was convinced that her unborn baby now had a broken neck too. She further believed that it was trying to get out of her body. If the baby remained inside of her, it would kill her. She had been trying to burn it out of her before it did her in.

Patty had not been drinking; nor was she on drugs. I hospitalized her because she was delusional.

From her records, I learned Patty's parents had died in a house fire when she was nine years old. Patty's pregnant sister had been awakened by the smoke, and she had managed to get the rest of the children out of the house before she returned to attempt to rescue their parents. The sister had been overcome by smoke and falling debris, and she also died. Patty's earliest memory was seeing her sister's belly pop open as her body was roasted.

Patty was sent to an Indian boarding school with her younger brother. Eight months later he was dead from a bee sting that had caused his windpipe to swell shut.

Patty left the school when she was thirteen and pregnant. She went to live with the boy's family, and after the birth of the child, his parents adopted it. Patty eventually moved out of the home and married someone else.

By sixteen, she was an abused wife. At least twice her husband was jailed for beating her. Following each of those severe beatings, she miscarried.

For Patty, everything that was lovable was eventually taken from her. If you believe that sooner or later some disaster is going to befall you, then the only control you have in that situation is to make it happen at your time, rather than to wait. That's why she stuck the matches into herself in the first place.

She had believed her baby would die. Another thing she loved would be taken from her. So she tried to make it happen her way and in her time. It was the only choice for her; she could never have given birth and then given the child up.

Now Patty's twenty-one-year-old husband was unemployed. He showed up in my office drunk one day, and he never returned. Patty miscarried while she was in the hospital. Slowly she began to get better.

She told me that she dreamed that snakes were coming out of blisters on the palms of her hands. Sometimes dozens of snakes would come out at once. When the blisters burst, the snakes would fall out and writhe about on her body. She would awaken from the sound of her own screaming.

Death was always around her, she said. Everything that she touched would die. She believed that she had some terrible power to attract death.

Just after the miscarriage, Patty feared that there might still be a piece of her baby inside of her, "turning into shit, to kill me." She tried burning holes in her belly again, to get the shit out.

I told her she wasn't trying hard enough to get her shit-baby out. I said that she must eat vegetables and high-fiber food to remove it. Then I bent over the broccoli on her lunch tray and spoke to it. I told it to cleanse Patty's insides with its fuzzy brush head. She ate it, and I prescribed a powerful laxative. She suffered from diarrhea and cramping, but when it was all over, she started to get well.

Milton

I understood this kind of stuff better after I had discovered Milton Erickson. His basic tools were always whatever the patient gave him, not just what he had learned in medical school. Erickson firmly believed that the doctor and the patient must share the same language and symbols and that they must together trust the unconscious. The doctor was only the guide as the patient walked his or her walk.

Milton Erickson was a maverick psychiatrist whose strategy was never to be restrictive and always to do the unexpected. A doctor did not have to know everything about his or her patients to be able to penetrate into the unconscious. In the proper learning environment, change could occur suddenly. One had to sneak into the unconscious mind with a message that it could hear: through indifference that triggers anger, through talking to broccoli, through religious or tribal ritual.

He knew that not everything can be explained. What's important in therapy is not direct interpretation; it's finding a way to get the person to pay attention. Erickson spoke in metaphors, in stories.

It has been my observation that many therapists avoid intervention with unconscious material because it makes treatment seem so simple. It is also rather frightening to assume that much responsibility, to trust your intuition along with your education.

Erickson wasn't afraid. He showed us that you have to use *all* of your healing skills if you want to do the work well. A healer is simply someone who helps a person confront opposing forces within him- or herself to promote health. Healing is accomplished whenever the needs of such opposing forces are successfully negotiated.

Erickson once said that the most important teacher he ever had was polio. As a child he was crippled, tone deaf, and color blind. He was also dyslexic. He taught himself to distinguish between the number "3" and the letter "M" because the three was "sitting" and the M was "standing."

Erickson insisted that you always make the best of the cards that life has dealt you. All people have things from their own experiences that they might use to see events and feelings more clearly. You are like your fingerprint—unique. There will never again be another you.

I had not learned of Erickson's theories at Yale. Even though at least twenty books have been written by or about

Erickson, his techniques were not taught there. They still aren't studied in most medical schools, now that psychiatry is moving toward a more "medical" approach that believes everything can be explained by biochemistry.

About a year before his death I met Erickson himself.

I had read some of his writings, and I knew that he understood what I was seeing and feeling in my work with the Indians. I was excited to meet this master who had already discovered what I was learning: to make changes, everyone — doctor and patient — must find his or her own unique way to fuel the creative unconscious.

Milton Erickson was in his late seventies when we met. I giggled aloud as I got my first look at his office, located behind his home in Phoenix. This rectangular add-on was decorated in vintage chrome and vinyl bus depot style. There were assorted ill-matched chairs, two-headed dolls, bones, dried fish, coconut skull with electric eyes. Erickson's wife, Betty, helped him into the study in his wheelchair. He was dressed completely in purple, the only color he could see. He sat there like an elf, a crooked smile betraying the weaker side of his body.

Milton looked at me, and I knew that my own smile of appreciation and excitement had given me away.

He leaned forward from his wheelchair and reached for a rock-sized piece of turquoise ore. For several moments he struggled with the task of picking up the rock. The process was obviously costing him a great deal of effort. I was spellbound, entranced with the silent drama of Erickson picking up a rock.

Then, while he looked at me and I looked back at him, he threw the rock directly at my crotch. For a moment I thought that I would be leaving the man's office with a high-pitched voice. Before I could react, the "rock" landed on me. It was a piece of foam rubber.

Erickson chortled and, in his Viking godfather voice, cautioned me: "Not everything you see is what you see it as. It is only how you see it at the moment."

Or did he say that how you saw it at the moment was really the way it was?

I was confused, but I sat there under his spell. Erickson was like a medicine man in his hogan. He was a storyteller capable of spinning magic.

Sometimes he would have his patients make pilgrimages to mountaintops, telling them to write down what they had seen and experienced during the climb. On occasion he prescribed ordeals, challenges that led people face to face with their monsters, their fears. These are the rites of passage into selfhood that many adults have never made. Indians have such a spiritual tradition, the vision quest. The purpose is to go to a quiet, isolated place and in solitude and readiness open oneself to receive what the mind wants to tell. The vision quest, like psychotherapy, is a transforming ritual.

Erickson could be a clown or a magician. He often used secret words, even fetishes such as masks and dolls. In Zuni legends, fetishes, usually carvings of animals in stone or shell, contain a spirit and will provide supernatural assistance to the owner. We use the same term in psychiatry to describe an object that a person has invested with magical, often sexual, powers. Clearly, such objects, in whatever way they become fetishes, hold a key to our unconscious minds.

Erickson never made a direct interpretation of symbols like fetishes or dreams. He was a master of enabling people to see their own symbols, to establish a pipeline into their own unconscious selves. He called this "strategic therapy," and like a skilled medicine man he helped his patients to maintain their own genuine, true connection to their centers.

Direct interpretations, Erickson argued, were an assault on the unconscious. The unconscious could find more ways to resist hearing something than you could find ways to say it. The therapist must approach the unconscious indirectly, even seductively, inviting it to reveal itself.

Repeatedly, Erickson emphasized that each individual was unique. Differences were to be treasured.

After our marvelous day-long session, I saw him one last time to give him a special gift, a Hopi Sun kachina, the messenger of enlightenment. A Kachina is a spirit, represented by dancers in Hopi ceremonies. Hopis teach their children about the spirits through the use of kachina dolls carved from the root of the cottonwood tree and painted to resemble the dancers. The Indians have many ways of keeping their centers visible.

At that last visit, Erickson and I sat together in his living room. The floor was virtually covered with Seri Indian carvings, lustrous heavy ironwood animals produced by a Mexican tribe along the Sea of Cortez. Before I left, he asked me to get him a leather pouch that was hanging on the door. It was a medicine bundle, the kind in which an Indian healer carries his or her most powerful tools. He unwrapped a gazing crystal and held it lovingly as I said goodbye.

Milton Erickson was a dancing healer. Herbert would have understood him, and Santiago would have applauded his dance.

Erich

A couple of months after Erickson died in 1980, another mentor, Erich Fromm, passed away. I wondered about the coincidence. Two months after Fromm's death, Mt. St. Helen's in Washington state erupted. Clearly, it was a season of change.

Herbert once told me that there would come a time when the seasons would change drastically. Summers would become unusually dry and winters would bring floods. There would be earthquakes and upheavals. Mt. St. Helen's, he would say, was a potent sign that the Earth was tired of its defacement by humankind. (Interestingly, the volcano obliterated a body of water at its base called Spirit Lake.)

The concern of Herbert and the other Indian traditionalists for the earth's rebellion was of long standing. In 1944, the BIA Hopi Agency had received inquiries from oil companies and other energy corporations about exploration leases for mineral deposits in Hopi land. At that time, the traditional religious leaders had written a letter to President Harry S. Truman affirming their position:

> This land was laid out for us by our Great Spirit. . . .
> It is given to the Hopi People, the task to guard this land.
> Not by force of arms . . . but by humble prayers, by obe-
> dience to our traditional and religious instructions. . . .
> This land is not for leasing or for sale. . . . Land is sacred
> and if the land is abused, the sacredness of the Hopi life
> will disappear and all other life as well. . . . Hopis are
> caretakers for all of the world.

Their case was rejected by a federal district court in Arizona, and the court decision was soon followed by the arrival of the oil companies, the explosions, and the digging for coal. According to Hopi prophecy, after such a violation of the earth, the state of order and harmony all over this planet would crumble. When the people couldn't follow the way anymore, then the Great Spirit would take the power into its own hands.

Erich Fromm would have understood this belief perfectly.

I liked Fromm and identified with him. He was a German Jewish refugee to the United States, a psychologist, and a mystic who once studied Kabbala with the foremost scholar of Jewish mysticism, Gershom Scholem.

Fromm was a founder of SANE, Committee for a Sane Nuclear Policy, an organization that warned of the danger of nuclear weapons. Like the Hopis, he feared that the earth and humankind were headed toward psychological and ecological disaster. In an age dominated by technology and consumerism, Fromm said, we are in danger of growing to feel more and more insignificant and uncertain about the meaningfulness of life. Fromm reached the simplest of conclusions: we must live by love. It was the only sane way to save ourselves from meaninglessness.

Once, I must admit, I viewed certain of these concepts as marshmallow fluff. But as I became a healer, I saw that people need love and a shared sense of spirit if they are to find a place to secure themselves in peace and belonging.

Fromm was a revolutionary in his own right. Once a disciple of Freud, he shed his mentor's sex-explains-everything libido theory, because he thought it a terribly confining position that didn't help us understand families and societies. Fromm admonished that society didn't place much importance on what was good for humankind. As a matter of fact, what was *bad* for humans did not make a whole lot of difference in contemporary thinking either. Toxic wastes in earth and air are the byproducts of the same genius that fashioned the labor-saving technology that we call progress.

The exploitation of humankind and nature renders us all out of touch with our feelings and basic needs, Fromm believed. Our technological genius entraps us and transforms us into machines. People hide behind masks of success. Though more of us have opportunities to amass wealth and comforts, we hide the truth of our depressions, annoyances, and unhappinesses.

Most people, Fromm thought, become co-opted by the demands of industrialized society for more production, more consumption, and more progress. But more progress in economy and technology does not mean more progress in people's search for meaning. The progress we have achieved is being directed away from the real spiritual and emotional betterment of people to an evil inner desert.

Fromm had no patience, however, with those who rush to embrace mystical philosophies to answer these dilemmas. He saw most of those as pure fakery and con-artistry, just more slick commercialism and salesmanship. Not everybody who said they had found the way really had. Using modern business methods, he believed, one could sell anything.

There was nothing fluffy about Fromm. He looked fearlessly at some of the truths organized religions and the healing professions often dodge.

Fromm is another healer who can help us get back on the path to pursue our vision quest.

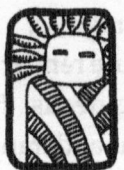 # THE CHURCH
OF FATHER PEYOTE

The first time I attended the church of Father Peyote, I got quite sick—and I was only sitting outside listening to the music. They passed some tea around. I tried it and became violently ill.

I thought that was the end of my relationship with Father Peyote. There was no way that I would sit up all night just to get sick. On that first visit to a Native American Church meeting in 1965, I did not realize that the process it offered was not to be taken lightly. It took me ten years to make a return visit, but now the church has become a place of healing and enlightenment for me.

To the believer, peyote constitutes a sacrament, not a drug. Peyote has absolutely no recreational aspects for the church participants. You must come to peyote as to truth, in an attitude of worship.

Let me explain at the outset that in matters of the Peyote Church, I am a guest who has come to dinner; that does not make me an expert on the entire family. I know what I have seen, and there is much I don't know. I go as a fellow traveler. I don't bring friends to observe the colorful ritual.

This is a sacred time to me and to every other participant in the service.

The most spiritual place I know is the tipi of the Peyote Church. I used to go to synagogue on the high Jewish holidays, but I can no longer feel the presence of the spirit in a group larger than forty.

Indians have a very different concept of where you worship. The whole Earth is the temple. Any place you stand is a church. The tipi is a nestling enclosure on the Earth Mother's breast, a place of sharing among a small group. Here each can worship at his or her own time, as the heart directs, in his or her own language.

I sing my Jewish songs in the tipi, and I wear my father's prayer shawl, the one he wore at his bar mitzvah in Germany. My Indian friends say that it does not matter in what language you sing; there are always at least two people who understand—you and the Creator.

The first time I sat before the coals in the tipi, I saw crematorium ashes. I do not see them as such anymore. I have allowed myself to become liberated. I understand that I am flawed and imperfect, so it's okay to feel small and weak. I am freer of the domination of those fears.

The more you work with the mind, the more you realize you can't know it. The more you seek to touch your spirit, the more you realize that you must enter some altered state of consciousness to burst free of the conventional limitations of flesh and rationality. This is what the Peyote Church is about.

I became interested in returning to the Peyote Church after I met a Road Man—a Native American Church leader, the "one who shows the road"—who asked me where I got my power to heal. I had heard that question before, so I smiled and answered, "I am still learning how to dance."

The Road Man smiled too. He told me that his healing power came through the sacrament peyote. "Oh," I said, a bit dubious. "I participated in a peyote meeting once and it felt more like a punishment than a gift."

He laughed and said that peyote's gift really depended on how you came to it. If you were a skeptic and approached it with fear, peyote would not reveal itself. He assured me that I could learn to receive the gift. This is a man I have since come to respect; we have taken each other as brothers.

I once provided testimony in support of passage of the Native American Religious Freedoms Act. From a psychological perspective, I testified, if the Native American Church did not exist, it would have to be created. I believe the church is one of the most important pan-Indian movements in this country. It offers a credible connection to something uniquely Indian. It is political, cultural, and spiritual—a source of pride, power, and psychological health.

The Native American Religious Freedoms Act was signed into law by President Jimmy Carter in 1978, but it has not yet been fully implemented. Although the powerful hallucinogen peyote is illegal to possess or use, the law allows Indians to consume it as a sacrament in the Native American Church, because of its traditional role in Indian religious beliefs. However, some states do not exempt church members from prosecution if they buy or sell it.

There is evidence of the ritual consumption of peyote as a sacrament by priests for more than sixteen hundred years, as far back as the Mayans. Legends tell that the sacred quality of peyote was revealed to a woman. One version says that a pregnant woman, lost from her band, wandering and alone, sick and weak, gave birth to a child. She was sustained by a vision that told her to eat the plant that was growing beside her. The plant was to be life and blessing for her and her people. She regained her strength, found her band, and shared the blessing.

The Navajo peyotists say that during the creation, it was the sacrament peyote that gave life, breath, and movement to Rainbow Woman, their birth-mother.

The Native American Church, as it is practiced in Arizona today, is only one hundred years old. It is commonly held that the faith came to the Oklahoma territory a century ago through Quanah Parker, a Comanche Indian leader. While living with his white mother's family in Texas, Quanah fell ill. When the doctors could not help him, the family called in an Indian healer; she cured Quanah with the help of songs and a bitter tea.

When Quanah recovered, the woman told him that the magical tea must never be taken for its own sake. It must be taken as a sacrament, with ceremony and respect. The medicine, peyote, came from the buttons that grow on the mescal cactus, and it was to be used for prayer, understanding, and healing—it was a sacred thing.

The healer showed Quanah the way to the sacred cactus and told him that it must be stalked like one stalks a deer—with respect. No one should wear the red mescal beads except during the ceremony and because woman first brought peyote to the earth, woman must always have a place in the ritual. She brought him to the meeting fireplace where he learned the ceremony.

When a healthy and fully recovered Quanah returned to

Oklahoma, it was a time of seething Indian discontent. The tribes were chafing under the confines of a neocolonial federal Indian policy that followed the bloody wars throughout the Southwest and Great Plains that decimated so many tribes. The Plains tribes were falling apart; the life-sustaining buffalo were disappearing.

Christian churches were springing up everywhere among the Indians. Their central myths were already familiar through traditional Indian beliefs. Virgin births, saviors, miracles, healings, and raising people from the dead already made sense, and the church promised salvation.

Also at this time Wovoka, a Paiute, introduced to the Plains tribes a new amalgamation of tribal religions and Christian elements called the Ghost Dance. The Ghost Dance was based on a hatred of whites and a hope of doing away with them to bring back the old Indian ways. Dancers wore cotton or buckskin shirts painted with "bulletproof" designs to protect the wearer. The vests didn't work, but the movement hasn't failed. Feelings against whites still bring all Indians together. The Ghost Dance is undergoing resurgence, as are so many traditional Indian ways.

Into this atmosphere Quanah brought the sacrament peyote back to his Comanche tribe. A vision at the holy mountain near present-day Cache, Oklahoma, ordered him to bring this sacrament to his people to perpetuate the ways he had been taught. Quanah brought the beads and the sash worn by the Peyote Chief, called the Road Man. He also brought the elements of the peyote ceremony: fire and cedar incense, the water drum, the peyote fans, the staff, the gourd rattle, and the smoking of sweet tobacco and peyote.

The peyote religion spread throughout the Indian world, each tribe adding its own variations. The Christian churches and government agents argued against it as the way of the Devil that transformed their Indian flocks into drug-crazed savages. But many of the Indians saw it as something of their own, a way to the spirit. The Navajo were introduced to peyote in the early 1900s, probably through students who were initiated in boarding schools. Soon tribes from east to west were holding peyote ceremonies.

This uniquely pan-Indian religion today may have as many as 300,000 participants. Many observers have found it to be the single most effective program to deal with the problem of Indian alcoholism.

The Native American Church has members from nearly every tribe on the North American continent. It sometimes incorporates Christian symbology in its rituals, yet it expresses the ideals of the older traditions: each individual is a part of the harmonious creation of the universe. With all things we are as brothers and sisters and must live together in harmony and peace. The Earth Mother must be treated with respect and gratitude.

The members of the Native American Church are essentially universalists, regarding all religions as basically good and variations on the same theme. They stress humility, faith, and love toward all and believe that a man or woman trying to function alone is weak. All must seek the Creator's guidance for true strength and redemption. Peyote offers the communicant a method of establishing contact with the Creator.

I liked the Road Man I met. He was not a salesman, just a believer. We talked about treatment failures as well as successes. He said undefensively that his failures reminded him that he was just one small cog in a much bigger machine. The mysterious was unfathomable. I knew in my heart that I was more ready now to participate in Father Peyote's church than I had been before. The Road Man invited me to a service.

We met at the tipi at dusk for a ceremony that would last until sunrise. In the enclosing darkness, people talked in small groups, and other than the Road Man, I knew no one. Then at nightfall we lined up in front of the huge tipi, which held more than thirty people around a central fire. I felt like a traveler to another place and time.

The taking of the awesome, psychodynamically powerful drug still frightened me a little. But I went to the meeting with a positive attitude, and the Road Man had reassured me that it would take care of itself. He respected the power of peyote and he had never seen problems. He explained that everyone had come together for the purpose of enlightenment.

It was time. We walked around the tipi while the Road Man chanted. Then we entered, following the Road Man through a flap opening on the east side where the sun's first rays would strike. The Road Man, also called the chief, sat at the west end, opposite the tipi opening. On the Road Man's right was the man who "carried drum"; on his left, the sponsors of the meeting. The other participants all sat on the earth floor on blankets, strips of carpet, or pillows. Because of my back problem, I had brought a small beach chair; afterward some called me the "Chair Man." At the flap opening sat the Fire Man. He would replenish the wood, spread the ashes, pick up the smoked offerings, and sweep the ground.

When all were seated, the chief opened his ceremonial bundle and removed the contents: an eagle-feather fan, a gourd rattle, tobacco and corn husks, a staff, and an eagle-bone whistle. In the center of the tipi was a fire with the logs placed in a "V." It flamed at its apex, which faced the Road Man.

In front of the Road Man was a three-inch-wide, six-foot-long crescent-shaped altar representing the moon, another traditional mother of humankind, made of wet sand. Its open ends faced the flap. After the Road Man blessed the symbolic items from his bundle, he placed his own special peyote cactus head, Chief Peyote or "Father Peyote," on top of the crescent altar on small branches of sage. Father Peyote was the focal point in the ceremony—it would keep us together on the road. It had been given to the chief by his grandfather. He told us to look at it, and it would teach us.

After his brief preamble, the Road Man had little to say. Each of us held the keys to our own path. The medicine would help us find our way to help the Road Man to assist us.

The Drum Man picked up his instrument. A rope and tiny round pebbles anchored the hide cover to a small, black, three-legged iron kettle half filled with water and chunks of charcoal. He drummed five or six beats a second. The drum music was strong, rhythmic, hypnotic, and I hummed with the beat.

We rolled the "opening smoke," placing sweet tobacco in corn husks. It had an anise-like taste and I coughed uncontrollably. Each smoker released a prayer with his or her smoke, and the whispy tendrils rose through the hole in the ceiling to the sky, taking the prayers to God. Fire Man carefully dragged some coals from the fire with a curved stick and piled them inside the crescent so that Cedar Man could sprinkle the cedar upon them as a fragrant accompaniment to the ascending prayers. All the participants blew and patted the smoke on to themselves. When we had completed this first smoke, we placed the butts on the edge of the altar for the Fire Man to pick up.

A bunch of fresh sage was passed from member to member, and each of us removed a few leaves to rub on our hands. Sage has traditionally been sacred to the Indian; the peyote people say it was the first plant God gave to the Earth Mother.

Then came the peyote—in a bowl, watered down into a loose cereal. (I have since eaten it as a dry powder, chewed it whole, or taken it as dried slices.) I gagged when I swallowed it—it was unbelievably bitter. Later I wanted to leave to vomit, but the Road Man told me it was okay to vomit right there.

Have you ever vomited in front of a group of strangers? It breaks down boundaries faster than anything I've yet discovered. No big deal. The Fire Man shovels and sweeps up the vomit. No one seems to notice, much less mind. The Road Man came to me and waved his fan over me as I inhaled deeply. He said it was supposed to come up, and here everything can be revealed without shame. I felt better.

The drum, gourd rattle, and staff were passed clockwise all night. We each had a chance to play them while singing if we chose to do so. In this ceremony, participants chant, smoke, and pray, and together create a catalyst for reflection. When worshipers finished their chants and songs, the Road Man sprinkled cedar onto the coals, and the sweet smoke rose animatedly from the fire.

After the first round of songs, Cedar Man smoked tobacco and prayed for healing for members of the circle who were absent because of illnesses. He asked a special blessing for the leaders of the nation, for the soldiers who serve it, for the sick and the poor, for rain, for crops, and for all the creatures of the earth. He beseeched Grandfather/Creator to bless the Native American Church, all its members, and all other people who want peace and brotherhood.

The singing continued. Participants took as much peyote as they felt was needed to guide them on their paths.

As the Road Man waved his fan at the cedar, I saw the black and white feathers melding into his flesh. His forearm became the wing of an eagle. I felt myself being waved upward along with the cedar smoke—I was rising out of my body. I became frightened for a moment that I might waft out through the top tipi hole. I was floating, looking at myself disembodied. I wanted to reach out to hold onto the chair, but I could not move my arm. I tried to speak, but no words came.

The Road Man saw my lips moving and the tears I did not even feel. He sprinkled water on my face and touched me, leaving his hand on me. "Look at the Father Peyote," he said. He refocused my attention and told me to stay with it.

The Road Man told me later that only the body is grounded. The spirit soars and tears speak. I have returned to that memory since. It has taught me how to feel small, to appreciate specialness in things ordinary, to be less serious about knowing.

An overwhelming sense of well-being came over me as I stared at the Father Peyote. The colors were incredibly vivid; the songs were unbelievably melodic; and the coals formed a sparkling, volcanic mosaic.

At midnight Fire Man passed around a pail of water and a cup after blessing them with special smoke and a prayer. All drank, and Drum Man poured water on his drum and shared some of it with the Earth Mother beneath his feet.

With the coming of dawn the night visions dissipated. The Road Man greeted the sun with his eagle-bone whistle and his morning song. "First Woman," who sits to the left of the Road Man, then got up and left the tipi. That night she was represented by the sponsoring family's maternal aunt, but sometimes she may be the Road Man's wife or a birthday child's mother. She returned with water, cornmeal, dried meat, and fruit. She blessed the food and water and prayed for the assembly. Without her prayers this night's ceremony would not be acceptable, as words spoken to the Creator without First Woman's light of dawn blessing would not be heard. This part of the ceremony sort of reverses the story of Eve, the fruit-bearing temptress who brought about Adam's fall. Here, civilization is sustained by women. At the same time, Fire Man fashioned the coals within the crescent into the form of the peyote bird, which carries the soul to God.

After our symbolic meal, the Road Man led the closing rite of prayers while he returned the peyote symbols to his case. The hide was removed from the iron kettle and the lumps of charcoal placed on the glowing coals of the fire. The water from the drum was poured along the upper edge of the crescent altar.

I stood to go outside. Except for a short break at about midnight I'd now been sitting for almost six hours straight and had no back pain.

Before leaving the tipi, people spoke of their appreciation for having been there. The Road Man gave his ceremonial bundle to the Fire Man, who carried it out, and we all emerged behind him, talking of the night's experience.

Moments of insight and new awareness—altered states of consciousness—can occur any time or anywhere. Usually we try to control the experience and minimize its potential impact by devising methods to cover it up or explain it, rather than appreciate or reexperience it.

My experience has been that if you feel it as real, go with it, and don't diminish it. Trust your unconscious; it will take you to a place of enlightenment. It is a part of you that usually guides you to a new place that offers nothing to fear. If you only see what seems to make you comfortable, then you are always destined to relive the old experiences and remain closed to discovering new levels of your own being.

In our culture, any experience of the intuitive, unencumbered, less controlled part of the mind has generally been repressed. Artists and others of creative mind know that the unconscious must be uninhibited to make the associations that produce new understanding. It is being open to the unconscious that allows insight to blossom into conscious comprehension.

Children are too often reprimanded for expressing their imagination, and soon they lose touch with it. In our culture the rational problem-solving part of our minds has become ascendant. But we must never lose sight of the intuitive, right-brain processes. Our obsession with what is rational is the most unfortunate consequence of a contemporary scientific attitude that reduces all "being" to a single dimension, to what can be seen, repeated, proven, and quantified by "objective" research and observation. Such dogmatism in the way we view reality limits our ability to open ourselves up to the multilevel states of being that may also have something to teach us.

Erich Fromm knew that our rational, scientific, production-and-consumption orientation closes us off from the other parts of our selves. Herbert knew that the mind is mysterious, and Santiago knew that to heal you must be able to dance, to hear the music from deep within. All knew that we are doomed if we don't follow the walk to our souls.

The Road Man says peyote is a messenger to one's soul. Now I want to tell you two stories about how Father Peyote spoke his message.

Chapter 6

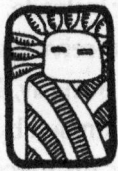

DELBERT AND BILLY:
TWO PEYOTE STORIES

Delbert

When I learned that I had an appointment to see a man who had confessed to the murder of a baby, I felt repugnance even before I met him.

A psychiatrist's opinions, like anyone else's, may be colored by his or her preconceptions, but we hope that our professional training can reprogram us so we will not be forever bound by those preconceptions. I made a sincere effort to shelve my initial disgust and to read the patient's file and the police report. They did nothing to relieve my repugnance.

Delbert had a rap sheet listing dates, charges, and legal dispositions that had begun in 1959, when he was twenty. He had been arrested more than forty times, mostly for drunken and disorderly conduct. In 1962, following a guilty plea for a burglary offense, Delbert was committed to a California federal correctional facility, where he had served approximately three years. Since his release in 1965, he had lived in remote Navajoland with his wife and seven children ranging in age from ten years to fifteen months.

It was obvious from his dossier that Delbert's substantial drinking problem had not abated since his release from prison. The record showed numerous "drunk and disorderly" arrests on and off the reservation. A mechanic by trade, Delbert had been unemployed for five years and was receiving welfare.

For a week, from a Saturday to the next Sunday, Delbert had been in Holbrook, Arizona, occupying himself by drinking a cheap wine called Twister. On Sunday, his niece Sarah and her husband, Pete, found Delbert drunk and took him to their home in Holbrook for breakfast, then to her mother's home. En route, Delbert purchased another two-dollar bottle of Twister. He spent Sunday night in his sister's house with her five children, together with Pete and Sarah and their two children.

On Monday, while the older children were in school and the adults were gone, Delbert began to hear awful voices that threatened his life and refused to go away. That night, he was unable to sleep because of the maledictions.

The terrible voices faded on Tuesday but returned in the night. Unable to stand the sounds within his head, Delbert ran out of the house, tearing off his jacket and cap in an effort to hide from the voices. He was convinced that unseen presences wanted to kill him.

After running for an hour or more, Delbert became exhausted and returned to the house. He woke Pete and Sarah and asked them to take him to a nearby tribal police substation so that the officers could lock him up in the back of the police panel truck and allow him to go through his drunken "fits" without injuring himself or others.

The couple took Delbert to a police officer's home about 1 A.M. But the officer said he couldn't arrest Delbert or take him into custody because Delbert was not then intoxicated. Instead, at the officer's direction, they took Delbert to the community paramedic, who gave him two tranquilizer capsules and told him to go to bed.

The tranquilizers had no effect. Delbert was still hearing the voices and was a long way from sleep. He moaned that he was afraid of himself because of the voices. He convinced Pete and Sarah to tie him up with a lariat and with belts. After tying him up and locking him in a room by himself, Pete and Sarah and all the children went to bed.

From approximately 2 A.M. that morning until dawn, Delbert continued to hear the threatening voices. Some told him that he would be better off dead, because if he got loose he would kill all the children in the house. Others told him to go ahead and get loose, that he would not hurt anyone. Delbert began struggling to free himself of his bonds.

During the struggle he awoke Sarah and shouted for her to get help so he could be subdued and prevented from hurting someone. Twisting and loosening his bonds, Delbert warned Sarah that if he did get free, he was going to kill someone.

Pete and Sarah gathered all the children and fled the house in their pick-up truck. In their panic, however, they failed to take their five-month-old son, who was in a crib in the living room. Sarah jumped out of the truck and ran back into the house to get the baby. As she entered the house, she saw Delbert break through the locked door of his room and lurch into the living room with a knife in his hand. Then, in horror, she watched him decapitate her son.

Delbert bolted from the house, still brandishing the knife. He chased several members of the family and attacked another of his sister's daughters. During his rampage, he suddenly turned the knife on himself and stabbed himself in the throat. Unsuccessful in his effort at self-destruction, he threw the knife away and begged the police, who had by now arrived at the scene, to kill him so that he would not harm anyone else.

The Navajo police took Delbert to the Window Rock jail. During the ride, he continuously heard voices telling him he was going to die. Once the police learned he was hearing voices, they took Delbert to the hospital in Fort Defiance where he was given a tranquilizing injection.

Now, as Delbert awaited trial for killing the baby, the authorities of the district court in Flagstaff wanted me to offer an expert opinion as to whether he was capable of distinguishing whether his actions were right or wrong at the time of the crime. They also wanted me to assess whether or not Delbert could have controlled himself.

Two weeks later Delbert arrived in my office, accompanied by federal marshals. He had a chain belt around his waist to which his wrists were handcuffed. There were also chains around his ankles.

It was an interesting way to conduct an evaluation. After all, I am a psychiatrist. People are supposed to share with me their innermost selves, in the hope of gaining new insight and changing their lives. And, certainly, they are to come to me because they want to, not because they have to. Everything Delbert said to me, however, could be held against him. The atmosphere hardly promoted open sharing.

Being asked to decide whether someone is responsible for criminal conduct is a difficult problem for a psychiatrist. According to the enlightened Ninth Circuit Rule, if at the time of an offense a person's conduct was the result of a mental disease or defect that rendered the person unable to appreciate the wrongfulness of his or her conduct (including moral wrongfulness) or to be unable to conform his or her conduct to the requirement of law, then he or she is not guilty by reason of insanity. Intoxication can be the cause of a mental defect, but since people choose to drink, most juries find intoxication insufficient justification for a judgment of innocence. Psychiatrists have been empowered to render these decisions, even though we invariably disagree with one another.

I once attended a training seminar directed at psychiatrists who provided expert witness testimony. The week-long course featured Supreme Court justices, appellate court judges, district attorneys, police chiefs, and some jurors from the celebrated trial of Sirhan Sirhan, the man who assassinated Robert Kennedy in 1968.

The jurors talked about listening to expert testimony from several psychiatrists who had evaluated Sirhan. After hearing a number of conflicting reports, the jurors finally chose to discard all the expert opinions. They themselves decided that if Sirhan could have so meticulously planned the assassination—knowing where to park his car, where to stand for a clear shot, how to negotiate the escape route—he couldn't be all crazy. So much for the expert testimony.

In my office, Delbert was alert and aware of both his present surroundings and the events that had brought him to me. He presented no evidence of psychotic thinking, no conspicuous signs of craziness.

Delbert told me that he had been reared in a sheepherding family. His father drank chronically, as did his brothers and sisters. Delbert had attended boarding schools from the time he was eight because BIA social workers felt that his home environment was not conducive to a healthy upbringing. He went home only for summer vacations. Delbert didn't do well scholastically, but he was excellent with his hands. He wanted to become a mechanic, but such course work was not available in the curriculum at that time.

Delbert told me, with sadness, that from the time he was fifteen years old at boarding school he had drunk heavily. He had probably been a chronic alcoholic since that time, was expelled from school for drinking, and had not held a steady job since.

During the last five years, he had been mostly unemployed, spending his time drinking cheap wine. He binged weekly, with or without money. There were always friends to share a bottle with him.

He stayed away from his family during these times, sometimes for weeks, until somebody fetched him. He had been in delerium tremens at least three times. These terrifying alcoholic hallucinations made him paranoid. Sometimes he didn't get the full-blown hallucinations and terrors—more often just the shakes and some perceptual distortions. On the night at his sister's house, the terrors had taken complete control.

Delbert knew he had killed his niece's baby and felt terrible guilt about it, but he didn't believe that he had committed the murder. It was the alcohol that did it, that made him do it.

Many Indian alcoholics—and their communities—look at such behavior that way—the drinker is never held responsible for his or her behavior while drinking. The abuse of alcohol is perpetuated by this tacit understanding that a drinker can say or do things while drunk that would be impossible to express otherwise.

My first reaction to Delbert's story was to look for some reason to find him guilty of his unspeakable crime. But as I listened to Delbert relate his history, it became clear that he was suffering from an acute alcoholic hallucinosis during the horrible night at his sister's house. I concluded that he was suffering from a mental disorder that made it impossible for him either to appreciate the wrongfulness of his conduct or to be able to conform his behavior to the requirements of law. Because of his history, his loss of connection to a sustaining culture, his years of losing himself to liquor, he had done terrible harm.

He felt himself somewhere between guilty and innocent; he knew he did it, but it wasn't really he that did it. But the law doesn't provide such a category. There was a plea bargain. Delbert was convicted of the lesser charge of involuntary manslaughter, rather than first-degree murder. He would spend more than six years behind bars.

In prison, Delbert met another young Navajo who had been incarcerated for armed robbery. This young man was visited regularly by a Road Man from the Native American Church. Delbert listened to his friend. There were few other people with whom he communicated; in Arizona's prisons inmates tend to band together according to ethnic groups.

Delbert was alternately fascinated by and skeptical of the church. He had been aware of it on the reservation, but although as many as half the people he knew were members, he had never been a participant.

The Road Man was permitted to visit inmates, but not to conduct services. He could only talk about the church and its traditions and discuss its precepts with the Indian residents. Delbert told me that the Road Man was a spellbinding storyteller. Delbert learned that peyote had been given to the Navajos at the beginning of creation, but that his people had not then been ready to receive it. Because of the Navajos' lack of awareness, the gift had been given to the people of the south.

In his first year of imprisonment, Delbert spoke to the Road Man about his guilt and shame. He told him that he wanted to return to the reservation, yet he was also afraid to go back to face the people who knew what he had done.

The Road Man told Delbert that he could follow peyote's path and seek a new vision, a new meaning for himself. He said peyote was a good way and that its power was a blessing to share among friends. Delbert felt so drawn to the concept that he knew he would participate on his release.

Six and a half years later, the Road Man sponsored a meeting for Delbert. That first night Delbert looked into the fire and saw his lined face as shriveled and old. In the green-flamed coals he saw the remnants of broken wine bottles.

The Road Man saw Delbert gasp, and he went to him at once. He waved his eagle fan over him and told him to focus on the sacrament on the altar. It would provide the answer. And Delbert knew that it already had.

He became a regular participant in the Peyote Church. He has never had another drink.

Billy

Billy and I worked together when he served as a physician's assistant on an isolated Indian reservation. For years he had been overworked – the longevity of physicians in this place was measured in months, not years.

Billy was the only health professional within a hundred miles. People figured it was his job to be available, so he was always "on call." He asked for relief, but nobody else was available. He asked for a transfer, but no one wanted to change places with him.

With no other relief in sight, Billy started drinking more and more heavily. One day when the pressure became overwhelming, he barricaded himself inside his house. Armed with an impressive array of artillery, he challenged all comers to try to get him.

I got a call asking what to do. I said, "Don't get too close to the house!"

I didn't know Billy personally then; but after hearing what he was doing, it didn't take much insight to see that he wanted us to take him seriously. I told the authorities to get a friend to tell Billy that we heard him now, loud and clear. We would find another place for him if he came out without his weapons.

The offer worked. Billy entered an alcohol treatment program. After the thirty-day in-patient program, he was reassigned to another job with the proviso that he attend Alcoholics Anonymous meetings and that he see me.

Being sober was a new experience for Billy. An Eastern band Cherokee, he had been raised in North Carolina by his sister. He had been drinking regularly since he was ten. He enlisted in the Army and got married at seventeen. Following his first military tour of duty, he had organized a country-western band and played all over Europe. He played, partied, and drank heavily.

When the wear of that life-style finally got to him, he had reenlisted in the service. He had been trained as a medical technician, and subsequently he went on for specialist training. After twenty years with the military, Billy retired to enter the Indian Health Service. By this time, he had been divorced and remarried four times.

The service desperately needed physicians' assistants, especially in the most underserved, isolated Indian reservations. Billy had been ready, excited, committed, and he had worked his butt off.

To talk with Billy was to be seduced by a hypnotic drawl. He was a smooth-tongued, country-style raconteur. Billy told me that he lived in a brothel as a boy and regularly endured the taunts of other children. He got into fights with such frequency that the authorities prohibited him from going to school. Billy had learned to play the guitar on a cigar box contraption, and he could sing the blues and those strangely haunting, mountain-hollow laments.

Many people who come to see me really don't want to hear what I have to say. A therapist's best students are those who already believe that he has something to tell them, rather than those who have to be convinced.

Billy was ready to learn. He told me that he knew something about sadness, and he was ready to give it up. He wanted to learn how to avoid more sadness. Through his sessions with me and his involvement in A.A. meetings, he was freeing himself of the alcohol that had produced his broken marriages, his panic, his life of sadness.

At A.A., Billy's natural charm made him an immediate winner. Billy said that he could "let his lip rap flap faster than molasses on a baby's ass." In meetings, he was confronted with an assortment of accomplished people as well as the hustlers, the frightened, and the lonely, and he learned from their stories.

Billy became involved with a new Universalist church and also with a woman about thirty years younger than he. He was still whooping and hollering in the western bars and remembering his old rodeo days of hard drinking and "buckle bunnies," but now he was drinking 7-Up or Perrier. He sometimes missed the taste of good "sippin' whiskey," he said. I assured him that I was appreciating it for both of us.

He was finding his own way, celebrating first a week, then a month, and then a year off booze. His relationship with the young woman moved him away from his preoccupation with his three young daughters, who had moved to Alaska with his estranged wife. Billy told me that he now had more energy than he had had in the last ten years. In the middle of this frolicsome relationship, Billy came to the office one day complaining of some difficulty in swallowing and a hoarseness in his throat. He saw a specialist, who said it was a little irritation of the vocal cords.

But in two weeks it didn't get any better, and after an X-ray he was told that something was displacing his windpipe. It looked like a growth that might have spread from his right lung. Additional tests revealed a virulent, small-cell lung cancer that had spread throughout his neck. For me, this was the first time that, in the middle of a treatment relationship, my patient was found to have an inoperable tumor.

Billy was stunned, angry, and overwhelmed. He steadfastly told me that he was going to "kick the cancer's ass." Billy read the literature and understood the odds. There was almost no chance he would last five years; most people don't last a year. Billy got on with the business at hand, meeting the new challenge. He was placed on a chemotherapeutic program and lost his hair. He vomited day and night.

I visited him weekly—at home when he couldn't move or at his little clinic, where he had joined a cancer self-help group. It is always helpful to talk with people who walk the same walk.

Our meetings were even more passionate and intimate. When you're dying, there is nothing to lose by looking at the truth and no time to waste doing anything else. It's remarkable how much you can deal with in an atmosphere devoid of bullshit.

Billy bought wigs and had fun with the varied hair styles—curly-headed wigs and short-parted coiffures. He took them off for the kids in clinic who loved to feel his smooth dome. He told them he was an extraterrestrial visitor. They called him "B.P."

During this time, he told me that his father had died of cancer. Billy also remembered that his father had attended all-night Native American Church meetings. Knowing of my interest in traditional healing, Billy wondered if he could go to a Peyote Church meeting; we talked about it at length. Then I discussed it with a Road Man and arranged for the two of them to meet.

Billy read about the church with the same appetite with which he had studied his disease. He wanted to participate, and I sponsored a meeting for him. On the meeting night, the tipi was full. I was there with Billy and his girlfriend—not as his doctor, but as a sponsor and a fellow seeker.

The Road Man invited us to explain to the group why we had asked for the meeting. I shared the fact of Billy's cancer and what had already been done to treat it. I said that he had asked to participate in this service because it was the way of his father. Billy said he had come for their support, their prayers, and for the energy of the Spiritual Source.

After the opening songs were sung, we ate the medicine. Billy gagged. He was chronically nauseous anyway, and the bitter plant was excruciatingly difficult for him to swallow. The songs, the drumbeat, and the fire were trance-inducing. The medicine always works well when you come to it in truth.

At midnight, the meeting's focal point, Billy spoke. He said that he had never come to the Creator in this way before, but that he had also never been this needy before. Weeping, he told them of his wish to live, of old ways and new hope, and asked for God's help. He appreciated their being with him now.

When Billy had finished, the Road Man told Billy that this was a good way, and in the way of peyote we could all find knowledge to help us. He would do the best he could for Billy, but it was not he who did the work—he was only an instrument in the hands of the Creator. "I am the servant," he said. "The master is above. But I will pray and sing, and all of us here will join so that our voices can be heard."

The Road Man walked to the fire. Poking around in the ashes, he picked up a glowing coal the size of a peach pit and placed it on a metal jar lid. He walked back to his seat; then, taking the coal from the lid, he placed it in his mouth.

When you perceive things from an ordinary state of consciousness, you see only what you have already seen. It is hard to believe the new vision because it doesn't mesh with what you think you know. Many of us find it difficult to acknowledge any visionary experience because of this resistance to new ways of seeing. The visionary experience shakes old comfortable realities.

The Road Man saw the burning coal from some extraordinary consciousness as something that would not endanger him physically. The coal spoke to him. That particular coal reached out to him and said, "Take me. I am the one." Using his cheeks as bellows, the Road Man sucked in air until the coal was white hot—we could see it illuminating the inside of his mouth.

Then he leaned over and blew heat and sparks right onto Billy's neck and chest. Billy sat unflinching, transfixed in the magic. The Road Man took the coal out of his mouth, placed it back on the lid, and carried it back to the fire. Returning to his seat, he picked up his cedar bag.

Dipping his hand inside, he sprinkled cedar onto the coals. He told us that the cedar gave color and smell to our prayers. We could see our words and send them on the wings of his eagle fan to be lifted to the Spiritual Source. The eagle is the messenger; it can fly high and serve as an intermediary between us and the Creator. His eagle-feather peyote fan had been handed down to him and he beheld its feathers now as if they were immortal.

"The eagle has faith, and we can learn from it," he said. It mates for life and lays its eggs only once a year in a place so inaccessible that there is room only for the nest. The nest is exposed to freezing cold and high winds, yet in this perilous place the eagle lays down its most precious gift. Our prayers should be like the faith of eagles. They will be sent skyward on eagle wings, to touch the ear of God.

At daybreak, the participants told Billy that they hoped their prayers would be found acceptable. They had prayed in the best way they knew how, and they too appreciated being there with him. The Road Man gave Billy the sage bedding on which the Father Peyote lay on the altar. To me he gave the bag of cedar and told me to use it in my prayers. I wondered at that moment what it might be like to put cedar down in the synagogue on the Day of Atonement.

Emerging from the tipi, we had coffee and donuts. Later we ate a big meal. Billy was not tired. His girlfriend, who had sat by his side all night long, looked pale and drawn.

We talked in the shade. Billy asked me if I believed in God. "Einstein was asked that question," I told Billy. "And he said that he believed that there was Something that explained the spiritual harmony of the universe. That makes a lot of sense to me."

The day after the meeting, while he was showering, Billy wiped a layer of dead, black skin from his neck and chest. He said that he felt stronger.

Over the next four months, he began losing weight. His time was getting shorter. The tumor had spread to his abdomen and he was in constant pain.

He wanted to see his children and his estranged wife, who now lived in Nevada, so he drove to Las Vegas to visit them. When his wife opened the door of the motel room, she involuntarily shrank back in horror. Billy, formerly a husky 200-pounder, now weighed 120 pounds and his face was cadaverous. The children called out, "Daddy," and he cried unashamedly.

He took care of final business, rewriting his will and visiting with his other children. Billy knew that I was planning to go on vacation in only a matter of weeks. He felt abandoned, but he told me that he knew I had to go. I too felt I was abandoning him.

The week prior to my anticipated departure, Billy was admitted to the hospital weighing less than 100 pounds. He was taking narcotics for pain constantly, and he lapsed into periodic confusion.

On the evening before I was to leave, I got a call from the family to come to the hospital. Billy had lapsed into coma. He appeared to be dying. Would I come over?

Should I go to the movies with friends as planned and then to the hospital? No! To the hospital now! On my way out of the house, I remembered the cedar and hurried back inside to retrieve the bag I had stored since Billy's Peyote Church meeting.

When I arrived at the hospital, Billy was unconscious, his breathing irregular. Around his bed stood a colleague from Nevada, one daughter, and his estranged wife. I sat by his head, held his hand, and told him that I had brought the cedar that had been given to me when we were together in the meeting. Did he remember the Road Man's instruction that I use it in my prayers? Now was the right time.

I repeated it as I understood it: the cedar smoke would carry him on his way to the spirit world. It would guide him on his journey like prayers to God's ear. Each of us around the bedside would add our prayers for him, which would accompany him with our love.

After closing the door to his room, I ignited the cedar in an abalone shell and brushed smoke on Billy, on myself, and on all around. I spoke some words and handed the shell to the next person. Each one brushed the smoke and spoke to Billy. His friend told him that he would remember him not as he saw him at this moment, but in boots and saddle, and that he would miss him. Billy's wife said that she would tell the children those things that would make them proud of him. His daughter brushed the smoke all over and said, "Goodbye, Daddy, I love you."

After all had spoken, I put the shell down. Then I turned to look at Billy and I saw that he had died.

Cedar is sacramental in many tribes, as is incense in Catholic and Jewish holy places. They have in common the holiness of smoke, the amorphous substance that wafts prayers to the source, to God.

We dramatically underutilize potential healing sacraments, whether they are rituals or objects that can mean something to us. The cedar that I burned at Billy's bedside brought together the people around him in a special way and enabled them to say words that otherwise might not have come.

I'm ready to perform sacraments with the door open now because I understand better that healing is also a spiritual process. Psychotherapists and doctors are priests invested with special power to persuade the spirit to heal. If belief helps a patient to find comfort, and if we believe we can help patients, then we must invoke the power of all healing sacraments to do so—to help the patient grow and heal, or even to accept losses and death.

Now, if a patient believes in ritual and sacraments, I put down cedar. I use feathers and herbs. It isn't that I have any magic; it's the rituals and their sacramental quality—they *are* healing.

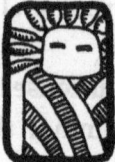

Chapter 7

JOLENE

The Mohave graveyard was a flat, stone-strewn field with few gravestones. In the old days there had been no grave markers at all. The human ashes, following cremation, were simply covered with dirt and left unmarked.

The end was the end; there was no engraved immortality. One returned to the earth, the eternal source, to become a part of it, to nurture those coming after. Previous lives, like the land, were a gift for unborn generations. Connections to the people who ended there and to the place itself could help avert disasters.

The Mohaves, a small tribe living around Parker, Arizona, are reluctant to talk to me of death and rebirth, not because I am unsympathetic, but because I am not Mohave. The few rituals that remain to them are carefully handed down to other Mohaves as an oral tradition.

In general terms, the Mohaves see dying as just another aspect of the life cycle. As in the creation myths of most religions, death and rebirth are part of an unending circle that connects all Mohaves with those who came before and, ultimately, to their supernatural ancestors, Matavilya and Mastamho, who created the Colorado River, produced light, shaped the land, and separated the Mohave people into clans.

I have also come to interpret death as the final adaptation to life. Death is when the body parts no longer communicate with one another in the old language. Death is an expression of what we once knew as life, but in another form. The task of healing, as I see it, is to maintain communication within the body as long as it is sensible to do so.

The Mohaves believe that when one dies the spirit is freed and goes on a voyage to the spirit world to be reunited with all its ancestors, a passage the living are not to interfere with. The body is only a container for the spirit, a reminder of this earthly life. If the body is not cremated, it becomes a burdensome connection to the earthworld and makes the spirit voyage more difficult.

Thus, when someone dies, friends and relatives return all of his or her possessions or attachments to earth. Toys, photographs, special gifts, clothing—all are burned. The deceased's name is not mentioned anymore. After the Mohave cryhouse ritual, tears are no longer shed for the lost loved one. Tears weigh the spirit down and make the voyage difficult.

I first met Jolene when she was ten. Her mother, Gail, a light-complexioned Anglo, and her father, Gabe, a full-blooded Mohave, were friends of mine. Jolene was a tall, bright child, an honor student who attended college on a scholarship. She was elected one of sixteen official representatives (the youngest of them) of the state of Oregon to the National Women's Conference in Houston, Texas, in 1977.

Jolene was usually active and striving, but while away at school she became depressed. She wrote to her father, who in turn explained in a letter that the forces of evil could sometimes capture one's energies. Jolene said that she wanted to take a break from all work and school and no play. She wanted to reevaluate and rededicate herself. She told her father that she wished to come home at semester break. She felt burdened, and she had dreams of dying.

Gabe knew of the unconscious, of self-doubt, uncertainty, guilt, and pain. He agreed that his daughter should return to recharge her personal energy.

At semester break, however, Jolene decided not to come home. Gabe told her to go and sweat—he would send her the sage and herbs to do it in the traditional way.

Ritual cleansing has been a part of almost all cultures. Christians have baptism and sprinkling; Jews ritually immerse themselves before Yom Kippur, the Day of Atonement. Indians go to the sweat lodge to cleanse the body and the soul before ceremonial occasions. To speak and listen to the Creative Source in the sacred grounds, you must get yourself in the appropriate frame of mind and be as cleansed and new as possible.

Cleansing is another ritual that has lost its sacramental quality for us. Now we go to a health spa and sit in the sauna or steam room as a social event or a beautification scheme. The native tradition, however, teaches that the steam is the breath of our grandparents and that the rocks producing the steam are invested with the spirits of all the people who have gone before. Sweating, with your ancestors breathing on you, has a healing influence.

We need to learn to separate the ordinary from the sacred, to learn to appreciate the mystery in small things whose origins we forget. Steam, incense, and smoke and ritual paraphernalia like candles and fire remind us of those mysteries.

Gabe wanted Jolene to go into a steam room and see it in a cleansing way. Then she would be prepared to receive the spirit.

She could receive her message by dreaming, her father advised her, and she should use the dream message to overcome the dark influences and help restore her balance. She had to do it now, while she was vulnerable to the forces of darkness. To let it go longer would only make it harder to shake later. He compared the dilemma to a hardening jello mold: you could not ignore the forces of darkness, or they would harden you. They had to be exorcised—met and conquered. (I think it not a bad definition of neurosis: the forces of darkness capturing and holding you until your "jello" hardens.)

He told Jolene that he and other friends would pray for her. My friend believed that prayers in any form, songs, and silence were acceptable to God as long as they were sincere. And he told Jolene that she must pray too. Her healing must ultimately come through her own being.

Jolene took the herbs to a steam room and cleansed herself as her father had suggested. She did better in school and was no longer worried; she became more involved in campus activities. The dreams of death dissipated, but she later wrote to her father asking that she be cremated in the Mohave way if she died.

Before the school year was over, Jolene was riding in a small car with some friends. The car collided head-on with another and Jolene sustained a massive head injury. The doctor initially said that she would not survive. My friend went to the Midwestern medical center to be with his daughter.

Jolene was in a neurology intensive-care unit, a fantasyland of life-sustaining mechanical wonders that overwhelmed

Gabe. She was unresponsive, but he sat at her bedside and spoke to her.

There was no way to explain why the accident had occurred to his daughter, no way to determine why it should be Jolene lying there in a comatose state. As we had often said to one another, "shit happens."

Gabe was a father maintaining a connection with his daughter even though she was unconscious. He was speaking with her as she existed between worlds and helping her to make a choice between those worlds.

In the old way, he perceived Jolene as existing in another dimension of life. She could see and hear things that he could not, but he could remind her of life in this dimension by telling her of his thoughts and visions. He spoke to Jolene of their home and his wish to take her back with him. He described the desert sage and ocotillo, the river and the sacred mountains of the reservations on which they had lived. He talked about Tempe, the house they lived in while he attended graduate school. He talked about her sisters, her mother, himself. He told her that in the place where she now existed she could still hear him and that he would stay with her.

Six weeks after the accident, Jolene was medically stabilized and, still unconscious, was transferred to Phoenix. When I saw her, she did not appear to hear me. Gabe assured me that she did hear, for he had seen her move her eyes. By the seventh week, Jolene opened her eyes. Gradually she improved, at first responding to words by blinking her eyes. Later she pointed to printed cards to indicate when she wanted the television channels changed and other simple requests. She still could not speak or move.

One evening I asked Jolene if she remembered the events following the accident. By pointing to the cards, she picked out her recollections. She did not recall the intensive care unit at all—she remembered hearing, seeing, and smelling her Arizona home.

Some weeks later, Jolene developed respiratory problems, and she was placed on a positive pressure breathing machine and fed through a tube threaded into her stomach. She occasionally appeared in respiratory distress, but her spirits were good.

Eleven weeks following the accident, she could sit up strapped in a chair. Jolene remembered more and more of the time before and after the accident, but not of the accident itself. She recalled visions of her family, her favorite haunts, the swimming holes.

During this time she developed a complication from the tracheotomy tube in her neck. A stricture had developed at the place where the tube ended in her trachea, but it was not seen as a serious problem. Periodically Jolene became racked with fever. She developed pressure sores on her buttocks. Her lungs became clogged with infection, but she was alert.

One evening Jolene tapped her head and pointed toward the wall at her feet. Her father changed the direction in which she was lying, moving her so that her head pointed to the north. The Mohave cremate their dead with the head pointed south. Jolene was not yet ready to die.

One day, Jolene was found in bed with the tracheotomy tube expelled. The doctors manually held open the hole in her neck as they attempted to insert another tube, but it could not get beyond the narrowed opening. A smaller tracheal tube was tried. Jolene did not complain, but she winced in pain at the manipulation.

While the doctors prepared the operating room for surgical reinsertion of the tube, Jolene suffered cardiac arrest. Three hours after the tube had been found expelled, all resuscitation efforts had failed and Jolene was pronounced dead.

She was taken back to Parker, where her family would translate her body the old way—after an elaborate ceremony. Jolene would be cremated.

For two nights before the cremation, members of the Mohave community gathered in the cryhouse, a white building that adjoined the cemetery. Jolene's casket rested on a raised central platform; the mourners placed mementos of Jolene next to her body, and one by one they stood and spoke of her.

The witnesses spoke only of the good things about Jolene. Whatever the bad, such shortcomings are only the baggage of an earthbound existence and should be left here, they said. The dead should only be remembered for their goodness, thus freeing them to rediscover their ancestors in spiritual harmony. Gabe stood and said that it was fitting for Jolene to be cremated in the old way, because it was a reaffirmation of the rightness of that way, an expression of life that could not be improved upon, an ethic about life that remained undiminished with time.

The cryhouse was filled with tears. The rhythmic chanting and soft moans in the background helped me remember the Jolene I once knew on camping trips in the pines, in Earth's peaceful tipi. I felt a giant ball well up in my throat, but stopped it there. It has always been hard for me to let go of tears; I still struggle to accept that part of my truth, that soft, vulnerable part that smacks of childishness or weakness or lack of control.

Relatives from the Quechan, the Cocopah, and the Maricopas came to share in the ritual. Gail performed the mother's ritual task of removing her daughter's shoes, a part of the tribal ritual she found comforting in her loss.

For everyone there, the cryhouse and cremation reaffirmed their way. Each person knew that he or she too would end in that place; and there is some comfort, I think, in being able to grow accustomed in life to the place of one's death. Death rituals are a useful reminder of our own mortality: your time here is limited; we must do whatever has to be done now. They also allow people to connect with the spirit and remind us that everyone comes and goes from this earth.

Such recognition and acceptance of mortality seem lost in contemporary life. One of the failures of current psychological movements lies in their inability to acknowledge that one day there will be an end to becoming.

As dawn approached, the pallbearers, friends, and relatives all stood as the casket bearers lifted the coffin from the platform. The singers led us all in the procession outside. When we had all emerged, the singers stopped to turn eastward and greet the rising sun. We moved again, accompanied by the chants and rattles. Then we stopped to face north, then twice more to face west and south. The stops would remind Jolene of the directions she had experienced in life and would tell the spirit world that she would again touch those directions on her spiritual voyage.

At the burial site the bearers removed Jolene from the casket and placed her in a pit lined with logs, a funeral pyre was about seven feet long and four feet wide resembling a truncated pyramid. The chanters stood only ten feet away, facing the brilliant rising sun. The rest of us, at a distance of perhaps thirty feet, formed a circle around the pyre.

From a large foot locker the assistants removed blankets, unfolding and draping about thirty of them one by one over the log pile to protect Jolene on her journey. Their bright rainbow colors were the colors of life, I was told.

Then, from inside the trunk, came old toys and dolls that had been returned to her in the cryhouse. These too were stuck into the pile.

Friends and relatives chose to keep only a few reminders, bringing the majority of Jolene's possessions to the pyre, so that Jolene would be completely released from this world to embark on her voyage. The Mohave concept of ownership eliminates wills, probates, and recriminations.

The chants became more intense. Our people circle swayed. In the early morning light, the draped pyre was wrapped many times around with a ribbon of bright scarves. The assistants moved back, as the one who bore the fire torch lighted each corner of the pyre.

A woman standing beside me in the circle removed her loose-fitting blouse and dress. Others followed suit and walked slowly to the growing fire to throw their clothes into the flames. In the old days, they would have cut their hair and stripped naked.

When they rejoined the circle, we rhythmically began a side-stepping movement around the leaping flames, circling in time to the chanting. The heat became intense and the circle moved back. The chanters came closer and threw their rattles into the flames. All of earth life relating to Jolene would be consumed.

The flames now reached twenty feet in the air, and the sky rained fragments of embered cloth like an anointing powder. I shuddered at the feeling of her presence on me.

We danced until the flames subsided. Then the circle divided. One half moved clockwise, the other counterclockwise; and each participant shook the hand of every other, then moved to the benches to shake the hands of seated family members. Shortly, Gail and Gabe removed themselves from the scene and then, quietly, all the others left. The crying was over. After the funeral noise, the silence was eerie.

The fire would burn and smolder all day and night. The logs, tilted inward, would eventually collapse, and the ashes would fill the hole. By morning, only a thin layer of earth would be needed to cover the pit.

Jolene's spirit journey had begun, and the magical intaglios that had been carved centuries ago at the bases of sacred mountains in the Colorado River Valley would show her the way.

After the cremation, I sat with Gabe and Gail for a while at their house. Gabe said, simply, that Jolene had completed her circle here. Hers had been only a moment in an unending spiral. All Indian life symbols are circular, without beginning or end. Gail said that her daughter was now released to choose again what to be.

All rituals, all sacraments are ways of preparing us for the inevitable truth that disasters occur, that "shit happens." Most of them are small when compared to dying, but one day we too will make our journey into another space.

If I, as a physician, cure someone and aid him or her to become less vulnerable to that disease again, then I am a good doctor. But if I, as a doctor, cure someone, aid him or her to become less vulnerable to that disease, *and* help him or her to understand their place in the universe, then I am a healer.

All the great dancing healers I have met have enabled their people to build bridges over the unknowable gaps, the mysteries, of our existence. They deal directly with the transition of death, and they participate in ritualized mourning. Then they get back to the business of living.

Chapter 8

SAM OLD DOG
AND HECTOR:
TWO OUTSIDERS

Sam Old Dog

Modern society, as Erich Fromm tells us, has many unhappy, isolated prisoners. In this context, I think often of Sam Old Dog, a twenty-eight-year-old Sioux Indian who had been referred to me by the tribal court as a wife-beater.

Sam had been a radio man with a Special Forces unit in Vietnam. After the war, when he was living in Phoenix, sometimes little things would trigger a feeling of being overwhelmed by aspects of his environment beyond his control, and rages would come suddenly upon him. On other occasions, he would sit silently and stare at nothing. Sometimes he drank to forget his misery and bewilderment.

His wife had become more than a little concerned that his erratic behavior would one day produce more than a beating for her. She feared that he might shoot her.

Sam was worried too. He felt bad about the beatings, and he told me that he had also taken to stalking road signs at night. He would sneak up on highway markers and obliterate them with a high-powered rifle that he kept hidden underground.

Sam Old Dog came into the world as a result of an out-of-wedlock pregnancy. His mother quickly bequeathed him to her parents, and they moved to Los Angeles when he was less than two years old. He grew up in the shadow of the Los Angeles Coliseum, the only Indian in a predominantly black and Mexican-American neighborhood. Sam soon realized that he was *the* minority in a minority neighborhood, so he was never certain on whom he might rely in an emergency. He learned to cater to both the blacks and the Chicanos by becoming a comedian. As a "crazy Indian kid" he came and went as no one's enemy.

Sam Old Dog's grandparents were quite religious, and he went to church with them on Sundays. When he was fourteen his mother remarried, and she took Sam back after his enfeebled grandmother was institutionalized.

Sam did not get along well with his stepfather. He spent most of his time on the streets with friends and became part of the California 1960s scene. He smoked lots of marijuana, experimented with hallucinogens, and played volleyball on the beach. Only once did he have a "bad trip." At an outdoor concert the popular LSD guru Timothy Leary was dropping rose petals from a helicopter. The swirling sawdust kicked up by the whirling rotors settled on Sam's skin, and he hallucinated that he was being eaten by bugs.

In the midst of this bliss, he received a draft notice.

Sam found a friend who had also received his "greetings" from the local draft board, and together they decided to leave the country. Setting out in a psychedelically painted VW bus, the two protestors planned to sell dope along the way to Canada to cover expenses. By the time they got to Seattle, Sam Old Dog couldn't stand the grayness, the cold, the wind of the Northwest, and he decided to return home despite the draft and the Vietnam War. By the time Sam arrived back in California, his second induction notice had arrived. It included the promise that if he did not report this time, a warrant would be issued for his arrest. Sam reported for duty.

To Sam's surprise, he liked the army. He loved the camaraderie of basic training and marveled at how skillfully the military changed men. First the haircuts, then the uniforms; everyone looked the same and had the same purpose. He also remembered Audie Murphy, World War II's most decorated soldier. He fantasized returning as a hero to parades and a nation's grateful applause. Sam was a good soldier. He now drank beer and smoked dope only occasionally.

After basic training he was sent to a front-line battalion in Vietnam where he spent eleven months surrendering and recapturing the same hill. His entire tour was spent securing its perimeter. This cyclical effort of capturing and losing the hill nine times took the lives of 60 percent of the comrades with whom he had arrived in Vietnam.

Sam described to me his recollections of sitting on the mountain at night when the perimeter lights went out, knowing that he was in enemy country, that he could die. For every day he fought, Sam got a day off. If he fought longer, he received more time off. On those days off, when he came back to base, he disappeared with friends—first to drink, then to smoke opium-laced marijuana, and finally to shoot heroin. Finding a woman became secondary. Drugs dominated army life, he said. Officers were doing dope just like the enlisted men. The stuff was sold openly out of duffle bags.

He was twice detoxified from heroin. The first time Sam admitted himself to the base hospital because he thought he had malaria. The second time the habit was heavier and the withdrawal more painful; he kicked it alone while on patrol on the mountain, gulping down great quantities of Valium to help with the shakes and the terrible feelings of desperation.

Three weeks after this withdrawal, Sam was involved in an action on a village. As he advanced on foot, air support dropped napalm. He saw a little girl run out of a flame-engulfed hut. She was on fire, so he took off his radio pack and ran toward her, but she was dead by the time he got to her. He stood staring, then dropped his weapon and walked back to camp. When the medics examined him, he was mumbling.

From the base hospital Sam Old Dog was sent to an area receiving hospital. He was psychiatrically discharged from the service as a chemical "brain-fry," a casualty of drugs, not combat.

Sam returned to the streets of Los Angeles. Though he had done his job in the army, there were no welcome-home parades, hardly even a hello. There were no jobs for soldiers who knew how to secure a hill in guerrilla country. Sam found himself unable to make new friends, and he lost touch with the old ones. He didn't belong anywhere.

He became seriously alcoholic. For a living he panhandled. Drunk or sober, he was still in Vietnam. When a Los Angeles traffic-watch helicopter flew over, Sam would sometimes scream and flee for cover under a parked car. On steamy summer afternoons, Sam could still smell the jungle.

At a bar, Sam met another Nam veteran who introduced him to the antiwar movement. He convinced Sam Old Dog that the only way his experience would make sense was to tell it to others who understood. Old Dog went with him to a meeting and became marginally involved with the group. It was not really his thing. He remained detached from women and continued to drink heavily.

Finally, after an arrest, the judge told him it was either jail or a treatment program. Old Dog picked an alcohol treatment program for Indians in Arizona. He was amazed to discover that the other residents looked to him as a leader. Indian country turned out to be one of the few places where being a Vietnam veteran was an honor. Returning warriors who had defended their land always received respect.

In the program, Sam also found a woman who helped him open up to loving, and they got married. Their relationship was good but sometimes Old Dog still had the dreams of the war, even ten years after his discharge. An added complication arose when he wanted his wife to get pregnant, and she couldn't. Sam blamed her; he blamed himself; he blamed the war.

When I first saw him, my barely suppressed feelings about the basic immorality of war kept me from being truly receptive to him and his war stories. After listening to him, I knew that I had confused my attitude about the warrior with my feelings about the war. I had avoided looking at Vietnam that way for a long time.

We talked about helplessness, fear, and rage, but it was not in my office that Sam got turned around. He anchored his center in his roots as an Indian and his pride as soldier, and he found those anchors through ritual.

Sam joined an Indian veterans group that participated in Gourd Dances, social events that are opened by a procession of modern-day warriors bearing the colors. Decked in traditional blankets, they affix their armed services medals to these uniforms. Singers around the great drum chant songs honoring warriors as they enter.

Before each occasion, the warriors prepare themselves by sweating. Old Dog described his first experience in the sweat lodge to me:

Twelve men sat close together in a small, canvas-covered igloo of willow branches. In the center was an earth pit in which hot stones were placed. The ceremonial leader lit a corn husk cigarette and passed it around and the men washed themselves in the smoke. The leader sprinkled water and cedar on the coals, and spoke to the rising steam:

> With this breath of the rock people, we will heal the pains in our bodies and our minds. This way has sustained our elders and it will sustain us. This way takes care of the winged creatures and those that crawl upon the Earth, those that walk or swim, and all that grows upon the Mother Earth. Treat all with respect, and treat yourself with respect. Our skin is the color of the Earth Mother; we are of her, and she is of us. If we remember these things, they will keep us together. Let us walk tonight with pride. We are warriors who carry the spirit of those who went before.

The leader then dipped the sage wand into the bucket in front of him and sprinkled all the participants. In the darkness Sam cried. The leader added cedar to the stones and the men bathed themselves in the sweet smell. They went in and out of the lodge four times. During each round, another member led the prayer.

When it was Sam's turn to lead, he said that he had never prayed this way before, that he didn't know how to do it, but that he wanted to say a few words in the best way he knew

how. The others encouraged him. Sam said that he was overcome with ugliness sometimes and that he was ashamed for
what he had done to his wife and to himself. The others mum-
bled their understanding and encouragement. Many had
been there too.

Old Dog kept going to sweats and to Gourd Dances. He
stopped beating his wife.

All sacraments offer healing.

Hector

Regardless of all the warnings in the psychoanalytic literature about self-disclosure, I now freely tell stories about
myself. I tell my patients Hasidic tales and Indian stories; I
sing songs and even make revelations about my own pain and
personal struggles. Of course, I choose very carefully those
stories that I share, but storytelling is important to my patients.
It is what psychiatry is about; you listen to people tell their
stories, and you tell yours.

The Indian worldview is pragmatic—you can't know anything until you've done it; anything else is a guess. If my
Indian patients are going to believe I can help them, it will
be because I've told them about the things that I have done,
not just the things that I know. This knowledge from experience is why you have to be gray to be able to heal.

The stories show that each person must become one with
the truth of his or her head, lips, and heart. If you say what
you really mean and you believe what you say, then you stay
healthy.

This is Hector's story.

From the time of creation, says Pima history, the Arizona
desert had rivers. Today there are only parched cracks in the

earth. The once-flowing waters lie entrapped in dammed lakes, serving the thirst of new desert cities. The Hohokam, the ancient ancestors, once dug canals by hand to trap the sudden downpours, so the precious rain could be used to grow food. Now rain water gets sucked into the dry earth within moments, or it floods the land because the river can no longer hold it.

In the old days the Pima were mainly farmers, becoming warriors only to resist their nomadic, hostile neighbors. Today they still live on their ancestral lands, but without much water. The culture and politics of the Southwest center around water. Whoever gets it thrives. Arizona's tribes are not doing well in this war either. They consistently lose to the cities, the mines, and the corporate farmers.

Hector's mother left the Pima reservation for Phoenix. Her first husband had disappeared in an alcoholic fog. The land could not sustain her, so she would try the city. But she could not support her children and her own alcoholism too.

When he was two years old, Hector was left with a blind grandmother back on the reservation. Three other siblings went elsewhere. Each day he looked at this gentle woman, with those clouded globes in her corroded sockets, and he loved her. She held him closely, and he guided her steps and picked up twigs whose bark she would strip with her teeth to make the baskets for which she was famous. "A blind basketweaver," marveled tourists.

Hector learned to weave too, while listening to her stories. They slept in the same room, on one bed. When he got older, he made the evening fire, tilting the sticks vertically to burn more slowly. He would later say that he had never known such peace.

When Hector was eleven years old, his grandmother died from the complications of long-standing diabetes, an illness that plagues the Pimas. Hector cried then, but he has not for a long time since. His grandmother buried, Hector went back to Phoenix with his mother. His grandmother had never let Hector return to his mother, out of her love for him, for she knew that her daughter was still drinking.

After Hector moved into his mother's house, he began some peculiar behaviors. He would stalk neighborhood cats and lock them up in a discarded refrigerator. After they had suffocated, he would hold elaborate funeral services. His teacher sent home a copy of an essay that Hector had written describing the evisceration of a baby prior to its burial. At this teacher's suggestion, his mother brought him to see me. Together we talked about death and dying and grandmothers and departures, and he seemed to improve.

After a year I lost track of Hector. But as a freshman in high school he reappeared when his counselor wrote to me asking for his records. Hector had been placed in a learning disabilities program because of his marginal academic performance, and the teaching staff wondered about his psychological status. Soon they sent Hector back to me.

The teenage Hector was nicely dressed and spoke well. He laughed about old dead cats; they were just a bad memory. He had friends of all kinds and was well accepted.

Then why wasn't he doing well in school? "Because of a lot of stuff at home." His mother was chronically alcoholic; among his brothers, one was a transvestite, one was retarded, and another was in the penitentiary. There was not a lot of love and no real home for him there. Hector wanted refuge, but I told him that it was all but impossible to find shelter for a minor who is neither flagrantly crazy, criminal, nor a runaway.

A month later he encountered the last straw when his family taunted him about his new girlfriend. He had fallen in love with a waitress and left her big tips. She appeared interested in him and promised to meet him outside the restaurant. He took his money out of the bank and continued to tip her well. His family found out and mocked him: "That white girl's just using you for a dumb Indian." Hector cursed at them and walked out, vowing never to return.

I still couldn't find a place for him. There was nowhere for Hector to go.

One week later he appeared in the emergency room accompanied by the police. They had found him wandering the streets, carrying a shopping bag and wearing nothing. In the bag was a pair of sneakers with which Hector said he would lead the American forces against the encroaching Communist invaders. The bag also contained a transistor radio, with which Hector picked up the enemy broadcasts and transmitted coded messages. Now I could hospitalize him.

In his dreams Hector reported being devoured by giant, sightless dinosaurs, only to find that he could live safely in their stomachs. He would live forever, he was convinced, because dinosaurs only eat vegetables. He became a vegetarian.

I told him that the giant reptile represented his blind grandmother. He wanted her to take care of him again. He wanted out of his world and back into her nest.

But direct interpretations, however insightful, rarely change behavior. I don't use them anymore, because people can find more ways not to hear them than you have ways of saying them.

In the hospital, Hector participated in a psychodrama where people act out what's on their minds within a group of people who can give input and discuss the individual's pain. A boy in the group talked about his prostitute mother; he wished that he had never been born. The group translated his fantasy into a whole production number and created a new birth for him: he could pick his ideal mother and be reborn.

While someone was pulling the boy out of a vaginal tunnel made of sofa cushions, Hector suddenly jumped in to grasp his arms and shouted, "Don't be stupid. Stay inside or they'll eat you!"

The group leader asked the entrapped boy which way he wanted to go. Others in the group could help him if he chose to come out, but only he could make such a decision. The kid decided to come out.

The others pulled his legs to help him emerge into the world. But Hector resisted, tugging at the boy's arms, crying, and screaming, "No! No! There is nothing out there!" When the others prevailed and the boy was "born," Hector banged on the cushions, cursing with rage at the group's stupidity. It was a real breakthrough for the boy, and it happened without interpretation or explanation of why he felt as he did.

Later, Hector acted out his own rebirth with the group. At the crucial moment he decided that he too wanted to come out. With that decision, he improved rapidly. Once Hector decided to emerge from the protective womb of his past, he released a lot of negative feelings—primarily his rage at his mother, and at his grandmother for dying. His medication was eventually stopped.

Hector told me that when he was a child he had been treated by a medicine man. He remembered that the healer had sung and blown on him. He wanted to see a medicine man again, so his relatives found one for him. I wanted to meet the man and go to the ceremony too.

Can one cure by breath and smoke? I had been taught to think seriously about even touching a person goodbye, much less sucking or blowing on someone. But I wanted to learn.

The medicine man, Francisco, was an old man—how old he didn't know. Francisco knew Hector's childhood story, and I filled in details about his recent experiences. The old man thought Hector had an insufficient life force to sustain him. His life force had been compromised, maybe even before his birth. His mother may have violated a taboo, perhaps touched some dead animal. She had separated her life from Hector while he was yet in the womb. (Alcohol can do that.)

From the Pima perspective, everything has potential power because everything is invested with energy—not only people, but animals, plants (especially mushrooms, cactus, corn, and tobacco), and even stones, from small rocks carried on one's person for their protective power, to large craters, canyons, volcanoes, or earthquakes—all are expressions of the potential energy of the universe.

Francisco thought that he could strengthen Hector's life force by removing some illness-producing remnant within him. I used to think this kind of stuff was self-deception, pure and simple, because my training emphasized that behavior was the result of processes inside your own mind. The thought of some kind of diabolical possession as a result of touching dead meat was just unbelievable. But I know that a lot of symptomatic illnesses are expressions of the violation of some taboo.

This concept of possession, whether by witchcraft or unconscious conflict, is what psychotherapy is about. All healers, including psychiatrists, strengthen people's life force by helping to remove destructive debris; some healers call it exorcising devils. I've discovered that this kind of healing always works better when you use more than words.

Pima curing ceremonies are normally performed at night. Although I work almost exclusively in the daytime, I know that in the darkness we can more clearly see the illusions, distortions, and ghosts that live in the imagination. I have found that holding groups at night, outdoors with a fire if possible, powerfully facilitates their purpose.

This ceremony was to be both a diagnostic and a curing session for Hector. Francisco and his helpers came together early to create the strength necessary to heal. They smoked the house with sage. The atmosphere was as if they were preparing for a struggle.

Francisco would "illuminate" Hector's belly by the use of feathers and fetishes and smoke so he could see the offending source. Once he could see the problem, he would be able to mobilize the specific positive strength necessary to counteract it.

Francisco and his associates approached Hector with chanting, singing, and the shaking of rattles. They blew smoke on him, sometimes bending only inches above him. Some blew smoke toward the chimney hole, seeking to push their completed songs and prayers toward the spirit world. Francisco smoked special tobacco and blew it on Hector, then retreated to the furthest corner of the house and waved an eagle-feather fan at the songs as they emerged from his mouth. He directed the songs at Hector and far beyond him.

Francisco rubbed earth and ashes around Hector's belly button. He waved the eagle fan over the boy and leaned over him. From Hector's belly button he sucked out some teeth. The medicine man showed the glistening, jagged pearls to Hector, and then the teeth disappeared.

When the ritual was over, Francisco and the others pressed their hands on Hector. During the next several days, they monitored him to see if the removal of the negative forces and the induction of positive ones would take hold.

None of this seems silly to me anymore. Francisco and I both perceived Hector's problem as one of maternal deprivation. I talked to Hector about his pain. Francisco removed the internal conflict more actively, just as the psychodrama group had forced Hector's commitment to life. All the methods worked together to help Hector in his healing process. He had been reborn, this time into health and life, and he could proceed without his old fears.

This is how I understand Hector's story. When it comes to understanding the mind, we are like children. Even if we someday know the brain and its chemistry, the mind will always have a mind of its own. The mind is a multifaceted jewel that snatches at whatever light comes in from many angles and creates a myriad of hues and colors. There are as many ways to see the light as there are ways to create it.

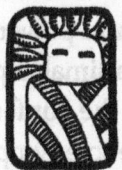 **TWIN BOY AND THE TOMATO LADY: TWO TALES OF WITCHCRAFT**

Twin Boy

I was conducting a seminar about human behavior for personnel at an Apache reservation hospital when someone raised the issue of witchcraft. Did I really believe, I was asked, that someone could make another person ill by casting a spell?

Most questions are really statements in disguise. There is power in everything, I say, as I have come to understand it. Objects and animals as well as people can influence human behavior. And witches can devise ways to influence your spirit. Witchcraft is just another attempt to explain things, a way of dealing with the dark forces that appear to have influence over our lives. I had come to believe that many things and many people could make us ill, because we are all needy, vulnerable, and to some degree, suggestible human beings.

Indian traditions have a strong belief in spirits and the healing presence of sacramental objects. Witchcraft is just the opposite side of that view; it explains the concept of evil. A concept of evil is necessary to give us a sense of right and wrong, a way of knowing how to treat others. It is the way a society survives. We all know that people can do things to hurt us. We may call them evil, despots, inquisitors, or enemies; sometimes we call them witches.

When you believe in witchcraft you also believe that you can get rid of the evil spirit. The task is to find a power greater than that of the witch; it may be a totemic animal, a psychic, a medicine man, a ceremony, surgery, or the confessional.

Curiously, I cannot always determine the sole symptomatic cause of an illness, so I really can't say that it hasn't been caused by a spell. But I do have a way to remove "curses" that have been set in motion by pain and fear. Furthermore, I told the group, I have discovered that I can remove a curse better by doing something to it than by interpreting it.

The process of psychotherapy is, in a sense, a kind of witchcraft made complicated. The therapist removes "spells" by assisting the patient to discover a power within him- or herself that is greater than the power that produced the symptom.

If I'm working with someone who believes in a system of good and evil powers, then I help him or her find the power that's greater than the evil one. If the patient gives me clues to ways of finding that power by using certain words or revealing certain beliefs, then I can use that context to help the patient win the struggle. It's what Milton Erickson meant when he taught that the symbols must have meaning for the patient.

After my presentation, a woman named Marti asked to speak with me for a moment. Could I keep a secret? She wanted to tell me something that nobody else knew. I felt her urgency and assured her that whatever she wanted to say would be just between us.

Marti began by saying that she had become increasingly depressed over the past two years. Night terrors would awaken her and she couldn't fall back asleep. What was worse, she believed that her terrifying dreams would one day come true.

All the dreams had to do with her youngest brother. Her sixteen-year-old brother, Marti told me, had been tied to a bed since he was about two years old. Since the age of twelve, whenever he was untied, he would attack others or claw at himself. He spat at anyone who came close except his mother. Guttural, snarling sounds were his only methods of verbalization. He was unable to feed himself or control his bowel or bladder functions.

I was overwhelmed by Marti's disclosure. She continued her story.

Her brother had been the youngest of sixteen children, one of twins born to a mother almost fifty years old. The twin brother failed to thrive, and he died within weeks of birth. Some months thereafter, this surviving twin developed a seizure after suffering a high fever. He had convulsions regularly, which the family believed to be the result of witchcraft.

A medicine woman told the parents that the boy's umbilical cord had not been properly cut and disposed of. Through that improperly prepared stump, someone had transferred into him his twin brother's sickness. He could get well only if his dead brother's spirit were removed.

The medicine woman performed a ritual cleansing of Twin Boy, then burned things to help in the purification and the exorcism. She tied prayer feathers to his limbs. The mother too was told to cleanse herself. She was to shampoo her hair with special soap, drink a special tea, and not eat meat for some time.

Twin Boy did well for a while, but his seizures came harder. By two years of age, he required physical restraints because he banged his head, arms, and legs against hard objects. His family wondered if his twin brother was still within. The medicine woman said he might always be.

Twin Boy was never still. He would bang his head and eyes bloody. His mother remained devoted to him, sitting and playing with him for hours, restraining him only when he became self-mutilative and punched or bit himself.

His mother pleaded with the family not to mention Twin Boy's existence to authorities for fear that they would take him away; and after his infant immunizations, he never saw a doctor again. After all, the fever had first come after one such baby shot. In a way, she believed that his sickness was a curse that Twin Boy and she must live with. If the medicine woman's cures didn't work, there probably was no cure.

After the restraints became necessary all the time, the mother spoon-fed the boy. Later she would simply put the food close to his head where he ate it without using his hands. He could laugh, smile, and cry out, but he had never spoken a coherent word. Over the last several years the boy's frame had become deformed. He developed a severe hunchback. Still, the family kept his existence secret.

Marti now found it harder to accept the situation. Her mother was getting older and sickly. If she died, what would they do with Twin Boy? Marti felt she had to share the family secret with someone who would not laugh at her. The guilt, the shame, and the anger now were hurting her.

I asked her what I could do, and unhesitatingly she asked me to go see Twin Boy. I told her that I would come, but that she had to tell the other members of the family about my visit.

Marti not only made the announcement, but she told them that for the last two years she had been having bad dreams — so bad that she couldn't sleep and had no appetite. These dream thoughts had affected her at work, she told them, and she found herself crying at her desk. Marti explained that I told her she suffered from an illness that could be cured only by acknowledging the truth.

The family's relief was astounding. It seems that each member had been waiting for someone to offer an end to their shared suffering. By the time I rattled out there in the back of a truck, they were ready to consider alternatives.

I climbed out of the truck and walked with the family to an outside arbor under which Twin Boy lay. He was tied by all four extremities to a steel-cornered bed. Even from a distance I could see his hunchback. As I came closer, he snarled and spat at me. His fingers and eyes were mutilated; his teeth were decayed. I was speechless.

In the house, I explained to the family that maybe the time had come to think about what else could be done for Twin Boy. If they wanted, I would help find a place for him. The family already knew what needed to be done.

When Twin Boy first went into residential treatment, his mother stayed with him. The staff said that she related to him with extraordinary tenderness. He never snarled at her. One day she tearfully told Twin Boy that she was going, but that he would not be going with her. She knew that he understood he would never see her again.

The therapists and caretakers at this particular facility are highly trained and committed to their work. They helped this terribly disturbed child to become more self-sufficient. He became toilet-trained and learned to feed himself. He learned to bounce on a trampoline and to walk. Twin Boy even understood the token economy system in the home, whereby he got tokens he could redeem for candy when he performed well.

After the placement, someone entertained the idea of a lawsuit against the family for child abuse. I testified that when we take steps to confront serious human problems there are many ways to dance. Not only was the family committed to Twin Boy, but he had irreversible brain damage, and their care of him had saved the state at least three-quarters of a million dollars.

Twin Boy's family did not believe doctors could make him well, and as a matter of fact it may well have been a doctor who made him sick. His illness may have been a complication of DPT immunization, one of those one-in-a-million reactions to the shot.

The family chose to face their problem and care for this child themselves for as long as they could and in the best way they knew how. They had asked for help only when the mother had become old and enfeebled. There was no abuse here.

It's true that if Twin Boy had been placed early in his life in a superb institution like the one he was in now, he might have been helped to develop more quickly and fully. But, I argued, generally speaking, for one this profoundly impaired, being tied to a bed on the Apache reservation with the loving attention of his mother was better than being placed in most caretaking institutions in the United States.

The Tomato Lady

Della was a twenty-two-year-old Blackfeet woman from Montana, whose husband had died six months prior to her seeing me. A Mexican migrant worker, he was following the seasonal harvests when they met and married. They had lived in a town just off the reservation where Indians are still called "prairie niggers." He had been killed in a car wreck, driving drunk, two months before Della was to deliver their first baby.

Della brought Tesay, the baby girl, to Phoenix to get away from drunks of every description, including those in her family. She was significantly depressed when she came to see me. She raged against booze and her dead husband. After several months, she began to emerge from her deep depression.

I lost track of her for several years until one day she rematerialized in my office, terrified, chain-smoking cigarettes, and telling this story.

She was living with a man who was good to her and her daughter, but she had done a terrible thing. She had spent about three thousand dollars of what little money they had to have a psychic take away a curse.

Eight months before, at a county fair, she had received a "reading" for one dollar. The psychic had said that Della was in danger of repeating old mistakes that could destroy her. Della admitted that she was struggling with whether or not to get married. The psychic said she had already told Della too much. If Della wanted more details, she would have to see her at her office and she gave Della her card. Della could hardly wait until that evening to call for an appointment.

The following day, at the reading, the psychic told her that two people were conspiring to destroy her. They had paid a powerful witch to curse her. But if Della paid her five thousand dollars, then the psychic could prevent this disaster from happening. Della was not to tell anyone, the woman added. If she did, then Tesay, her daughter, might die.

"Bring part of the money to our next appointment, and also bring a tomato that you have rubbed all over your body," the psychic told her.

Della withdrew over a thousand dollars from the bank as an initial installment on the curse removal program. At her next visit to the psychic, the woman placed the tomato on a white handkerchief. She ordered Della to lay the large-denomination bills crosswise underneath it, then asked her to examine the tomato to see that there were no marks or blemishes on it.

After Della had completed the inspection, the psychic knotted the handkerchief and chanted over the bundle for God to help lift the curse from Della. She opened the bundle and had Della again confirm that there were no marks on the tomato. Then she split open the tomato. Inside was small, wooden head with real human hair. Blood dripped from its eyes and mouth.

As Della screamed in fear, the psychic asked if she wanted that to happen to her. "You must visit me regularly. I can make the curse disappear."

Not wishing to provoke such power further, Della began forking over payments on biweekly visits until she had given the psychic three thousand dollars, almost all that she had. When she finally told her boyfriend of the terrible dilemma, he was flabbergasted. He tried to sympathize with Della's fears, but his sympathy did not extend to his wallet. He adamantly refused to allow her to give the psychic another dime.

That was when Della came to me. She was terrified that the Tomato Lady had the power to seek retribution for her failure to complete her payments.

And what of the curse? Could that be reactivated against her? And now that she had told her boyfriend and me about the Tomato Lady, would the Tomato Lady make some disaster befall Tesay, as she had threatened? In desperation, Della asked me if I had a power greater than that of the psychic.

"Yes," I told her. "I have a power. You have power too."

Before she could puzzle that through, I shouted at her: "Give me your car keys! Right now. Give them here!"

Della was surprised by my sudden outburst. "Give you my keys?" she asked. "Why should I give you my keys?"

"I want your car!" I screamed. "Give me your keys!"

"But . . ."

"Don't question me!" I scowled at her. "Do as I tell you."

Although she seemed genuinely frightened by my strange behavior, Della stood her ground. "Why should I give you my keys?"

After a long silence, I asked, "Why did you give your keys to the Tomato Lady?"

In Della's confusion, I continued: "Not your *car* keys. But you gave her the keys to your personal power. The greatest power we have is the power to make choices. If you give someone the keys to your car, then you can't complain where they drive it. If you give someone the keys of responsibility for your happiness, then you can't complain if they don't make you happy."

How do we get the power to choose? We take it. It's almost as easy to exercise that power as it is to give it away. Doctors are vehicles for self-empowerment.

Indians try to look into the heart of a doctor to decide whether or not to come to him or her. The doctor must convince them that he or she has the power to heal. To accomplish this, the doctor must learn the many ways one can change the ordinary into the mystical, not just the opposite.

The melody you sing, like the steps you dance, is less important than the power of the connection your song establishes. The connection helps the patient heal. Della invested me with more power to heal than the Tomato Lady had power to harm. I was able to help her regain her own power. It doesn't matter how you do it, only that you do it.

Chapter 10

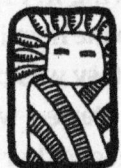

A KIDNAPPING
AND PAGE: CHILDREN

A Kidnapping

"Newborn Infant Kidnapped!"

The newspaper reported that a baby had been abducted from the Tuba City Indian Hospital in northern Arizona. A two-day-old male infant had disappeared, and someone had been seen walking out of the hospital with him. When they found the perpetrator two days later, she quickly admitted her guilt. The public defender sent her to see me, in hopes of establishing an insanity defense.

Dorothy, the young woman who had taken the baby, had been born to a mother who had not wanted her. She still did not know who her father was. As an infant, Dorothy had been given to her grandmother, who raised her in a small traditional village. She saw her mother rarely, and when she did come, her mother always referred to Dorothy as a sister. In the Navajo way, this rejection was serious and it always reminded Dorothy that she was unwanted.

But her grandmother loved her. She taught Dorothy to cook, weave, and participate in ceremonies, and the two of them became very close. When she was fourteen, Dorothy decided to get married, which is not so unusual in traditional

Navajoland after one boy keeps coming around regularly. From the earliest days of the marriage, Dorothy wanted a baby, but she could not get pregnant.

Six years after her marriage and now living in Phoenix, Dorothy learned during an outpatient visit to the hospital that she was pregnant for the first time. Her ecstasy was beyond words. She bought maternity clothes and started wearing them just to show everyone the wonderfulness of her condition. Her husband was as delighted as she. At last she would have her baby, and she would give it all that she wished had been given to her.

Five months into the pregnancy, in midwinter, her grandmother became ill and asked Dorothy for help. There was no way that Dorothy could deny the one person who had always been kind to her. She returned to the reservation to chop wood, help haul hay, and fetch groceries for her grandmother.

On the second night there, Dorothy awoke with cramping in her abdomen. She rushed to the bathroom and was horrified to discover that she had miscarried. In her hand, she held the precious but now deceased male fetus.

Dorothy crept out into the night and buried the fetus under a tree in the old way. The next morning she continued her errands. She met some relatives, but she told no one what had happened.

As she drove back to Phoenix a couple of days later, Dorothy's head was filled with one thought: she couldn't go home without a baby. What would she say to her husband? Did the miscarriage mean she was unable ever to be a mother? Why was she being deprived of this one thing that she so desperately wanted and deserved?

Dorothy had to come home with a baby. She could not think about anything else. In Flagstaff she bought some clothing for a baby and a striped blouse for herself. She made a plan that, in her obsessed state of mind, made perfect sense.

Dorothy drove on to the hospital in Tuba City. There she learned the names of some new mothers and chose one who had just given birth to a son. Wearing a candy-striped blouse and claiming to be a photographer's assistant, Dorothy asked the woman if she wanted some pictures taken of the baby. When the mother agreed, Dorothy picked the baby up from the mother's side and left the room. She kept walking to her pickup truck and drove off. That simply, Dorothy had her baby. She stopped to buy bottled formula, then continued to Phoenix.

At home, her husband and friends marveled at how big the baby was for such a short gestation, but a spirit of celebration prevailed. They bought clothes, gave the baby a name, and proudly showed him off. For two days, everyone could see that Dorothy was at last a mother. Later she learned that the name she and her husband gave the child was quite close to what the biological parents named him.

After her arrest and evaluation, Dorothy was released on her own recognizance. Her family held a ceremony for her. Everyone in her extended family was willing to share some responsibility toward the resolution of the event. In the Navajo way, when something bad happens to someone in a family or clan, it casts a pall over all the members, which the relatives then marshal forces to get rid of. This tradition is a classic example of community psychiatry, or family therapy, or systems therapy, whatever you want to call it. All promote the idea of bringing many forces together to best mobilize the powers that promote health.

Dorothy knew that she was not alone when her natural mother came to her during the ceremony and, for the first time, called her "daughter." At the baby's christening, his biological family prayed for forgiveness for the kidnapper, and then invited her to be godparent to the child. In this way, they offered forgiveness. Later, the child's family asked Dorothy and her people to join them on Mother's Day. They went, bringing a slaughtered sheep to share.

By the time Dorothy's case came to trial, both parties were satisfied with the healing and forgiveness the families had made possible. My testimony explained that both parties understood that unconscious forces controlled Dorothy's mind at the time of the kidnapping, and that at that moment she was powerless to do otherwise. She did not have a criminal mind and there was little likelihood that such an act would happen again. The charge was reduced to burglary. Dorothy was given a probationary term.

The families had made peace, and Dorothy had begun to find, through her family's love, a power that could balance the strength of her desire for a child. We could learn something from their experience.

Page

Kee and Desbah's six-month-old son had developed meningitis. On their way to the hospital in Page, they stopped to participate in an all-night ceremony — maybe a medicine man could cure him. But after the ceremony the baby was still in respiratory distress, so they continued their journey to Page. They planned to call a pediatrician they had once visited there.

In the emergency room, their doctor's associate was on duty and he examined the baby. Seeming annoyed by their presence, he scowled at the couple and pointedly asked them why they had not come to the hospital sooner. Kee and Desbah felt uneasy at the doctor's unfriendly reception, but they answered truthfully that they had stopped on the way to see a medicine man.

The doctor went into a rage. The two Navajos could not have angered him more if they had announced their memberships in a lobby for socialized medicine or in a cult whose members drank the blood of humans. "It will be your fault if your child dies!" he exploded. "You should have come sooner!"

Kee and Desbah literally staggered from this accusation as if the doctor had physically struck them. Navajo parents do not kill their sick children. The very thought was incomprehensible to them.

They left the child at the hospital, but the following morning they came to request the doctor to transfer the case to another physician; they didn't think this angry man could help their child. The doctor refused to see them.

Kee and Desbah felt they had only one choice—they must take their baby out of this hospital.

A nurse called the doctor and told him that the parents intended to remove the patient from hospital care. She hung up the phone and looked at them. "The doctor told me to tell you that your baby will die without the medicines of the hospital," the nurse told Kee and Desbah. "He says that you must leave the baby here."

"We have no choice," Kee told the nurse.

Desbah added firmly, "The doctor does not feel good about us. How can he feel good about our baby? We will take our child to the Indian hospital in Tuba City."

On the way to the Indian hospital, Kee and Desbah stopped again at the house of the medicine man for a blessing. He looked at the child and told them to take him straight to the hospital. By the time they arrived, their baby was dead.

Criminal charges of involuntary manslaughter were filed against Kee and Desbah. The doctor at Page testified that, in his opinion, the parents were responsible for the death of their child.

During his deposition, the doctor was asked if, when he first saw the parents in the emergency room, he had said hello or introduced himself. He could not remember. He was then asked if he had told them that it would be their fault if the baby died. He did remember that. He also conceded that he was angry and it had probably showed.

With the help of an interpreter, the parents told the court that they believed healing required the proper spirit. There had to be mutual trust among the healer, patient, and family. The doctor had not inspired their trust; he had humiliated them and implied that they would harm their child. They believed their baby would not survive in his hands. When he had refused to speak with them, they felt they had no other choice.

In my deposition, I explained that from the Navajo perspective it is unthinkable for any healer to believe that he or she alone does the healing. All parties—the spiritual source, the family, the clan, the patient and the medicine man—were participants in the healing process. To overemphasize one's singular importance and to denigrate that of others did not inspire confidence. This doctor blamed the family for their baby's condition; how could they believe in his healing power?

The case was eventually dropped. Hoping to avert a similar tragedy in the future, I wrote to the doctor and the hospital administration, offering to talk, free of charge, about traditional healing practices. In part, my letter stated:

> From the Navajo perspective, healing is a shared responsibility between patient and doctor. There must be a sense of commitment, belief, and harmony among all parties. Your experience with one another deemphasized such a harmonious exchange. It was a relationship of inequality in which the parents believed themselves humiliated. Hurt and angry, they returned to their own people and healers.
>
> Page lies in the midst of Navajo country and serves a large Indian population. The degree to which we can sensitize ourselves to the needs and beliefs of our constituents, even if we do not share those beliefs, will determine how we might better provide for their health needs.

I never received a response.

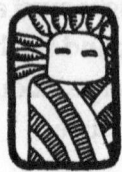

Chapter 11

POPEYE AND SOLOHO

The White Mountains of Arizona contain some of the most beautiful natural scenery in the world. Trout-filled streams cross meadows; forests of ponderosa pine lead to snow-capped peaks. The land sustains elk, bear, and mountain lion. The White Mountain Apaches own and operate a popular ski resort and a profitable lumber mill.

The name "Apache" conjures up silver-screen images of warriors in breechcloths, of cavalry forts and wily Geronimo. This is a people with whom the United States government only made peace in the 1900s. They are the last defeated Indian nation in this country, and they fought almost to the last man to keep their freedom. The concept of a reservation was entirely foreign to the wandering Apaches, who traveled over the hills and canyons of southeastern Arizona in hunting and warring bands of twenty or thirty people. Today's Apaches are quite disconnected from that colorful past. Nothing has replaced those old ways to give the Apache the same sense of pride and power.

I once asked a group of three- and four-year-old Indian Head Start students to draw a picture of their community. The children drew the usual houses, streets, stores, and schools. Interspersed among the buildings were stick figures. When I asked what the stick figures were doing, the children said, "Those are people lying around."

"What are they doing?" I asked.

The children answered, "They're drunk."

Even by the age of three, children accept this prevalence of alcoholism as ordinary. Alcohol, not the cavalry, may sow the final seeds of extinction among the Apache.

Whiteriver, in the heart of the White Mountains, is Popeye's home. Born to a mother who died of liver failure when he was a year old, Popeye was adopted by a white family and left the reservation.

He had a happy childhood and loved his family. Popeye got his nickname because he clapped his hands and gurgled when he heard the cartoon's theme song on television. He had a natural instinct for music. From early on, he banged rhythmically on any available surface or hummed with the windshield wipers. He learned to play the guitar, and he wrote songs.

In adolescence, Popeye joined the high-school Indian Club as he began to sort out his own identity issues. Although his parents openly dealt with his being Indian, they were unable to help him understand how it fit into who he was.

Popeye wanted to know about his biological mother. The adoption agency that had placed him gave him his mother's name, and he began to seek out what he could learn about her. On the reservation he met relatives who welcomed him back. As they offered him a beer, they told him about his mother's alcoholic death. Popeye spent some time with his relatives, but the drinking on the reservation was so overwhelming that he had to leave.

In his early twenties Popeye married his high-school sweetheart, a non-Indian. They had two sons, and he named each after an Apache chieftain. Popeye was proud of being Apache, and he wanted his sons to be proud too. He played guitar professionally while attending a local community college. The pace destroyed his marriage, he said later; he was just never around.

When I met Popeye, he was thirty years old and quadraplegic. This is how it happened.

At a party at a condominium, Popeye had gotten drunk and climbed onto a balcony that overlooked a central swimming pool. When he had everyone's attention, he announced that he was going to dive into the water. He did—and they had to drag him out. By the time the medics came, Popeye was barely breathing—another alcohol-related trauma, one of the so many Indian hospitals are besieged with.

A month later, when I first saw Popeye, he was depressed and withdrawn. He communicated only by screaming, primarily at the nurses. I said that I had come because the staff was concerned about how foul-mouthed and angry he was. He told me he didn't need a fucking shrink, and the litany began—"Bastard . . . fucker . . . white man . . . let me die! . . . The nurses stink . . . the government sucks . . ." and so on.

I went to my office to get a tape recorder and brought it back to his room. Popeye started his rap as soon as I hit the door. I switched the recorder on and left again. Fifteen minutes later I returned and replayed the tape for him. When the recording of his obscenities was over, Popeye screamed, "I hope you die. Because if you don't, I'll kill you!"

I yelled back. "Bullshit! It's just easier to get angry than to be afraid." I'd been there. Then I left.

Popeye stayed angry, but we talked. When he noticed movement in his shoulder, he started to mellow. A little later there was action in his arms and even his fingers and wrist. Now he wondered if he could beat it, how soon he could walk.

Popeye's attitude changed completely. No longer bitter and angry, he started talking about getting his fingers into better shape; he was going to make it in the music business. Now Popeye was laughing all the time, teasing the nurses, and talking about a marathon run.

I got suspicious. Was he denying reality and setting himself up for real disappointment?

I wanted to help him become more realistic about his crippled condition, so I asked him if he ever got mad or sad anymore.

"Yeah. I get mad whenever somebody reminds me that I'll spend the rest of my life in this goddamn wheelchair!"

A speechless moment. To me, Popeye's positive talk was not realistic. But so what? It was his life. My perception of reality is not necessarily the way it is. It's only the way I see it; it's just real for me. I didn't ask him to look at it my way again, not even when he told me he was going to be a marathoner.

For a long time I believed if you felt good because you were denying or minimizing realities, such feelings were based on illusions. Sooner or later the truth would come out, and you would be shattered along with your illusions. But there is intrinsic value to positive feelings, and I've learned that it's more effective to influence others using their perceptions of reality. I no longer tell patients how I see their reality unless they ask—and then I do so with considerable caution.

Psychologists using sophisticated tests have recently rediscovered this obvious fact: people who respond to a life-threatening illness with denial have a much better chance of surviving it. In all healing, the patient has a powerful impact on making it happen. Feeling or doing something positive can influence the outcome.

States of consciousness and awareness have a strong impact on the healing process. Current concepts of disease don't explain how, but these states can produce a change in one's level of physical functioning. Laughter can produce curative substances in the body; relaxation can lower blood pressure, increase blood flow, and raise skin temperature. You can change you brain rhythms; you can alter your perceptions of pain.

Science doesn't quite explain how this happens, but as a culture we share an urge for explanations. Indian healers understand that the questions are more important than the answers.

Herbert had introduced me to Bill Dalton, a Hopi healer, who lived in Whiteriver. It was from Bill that Herbert got his medicines. Bill had a controversial history and he seemed to have his share of detractors, but as he got older people sought him out. He liked to introduce himself by his Indian name, Soloho, the Whistling Arrow.

Bill's single-room cabin on the reservation was just large enough for a bed, a table, a wood-burning stove, and a foot locker filled with herbs. He was then in his seventies—vigorous, crinkled, a good-looking, good-humored old man who wore a headband over pageboy bangs.

When I met him he was skinning a mountain lion that had been deposited at his doorstep by the tribal trapper. After the greeting, I watched him, and he asked if I wanted a piece. It wasn't kosher, I told him, and he laughed and said

I couldn't use it anyway because it was more pussy than I could handle.

Years later, Bill told me about an experience in Hawaii where he treated a well-known singer who, for some reason, had been unable to perform. After Bill "worked on" him, he was able to go on stage that night. The story was publicized in the local paper, and some kahunas, native Hawaiian healers, invited him to attend a ceremony.

Not knowing what to expect, Bill went to the location. The kahunas blindfolded him and eventually led him up a mountainside into a cave where the blindfold was removed. Bill saw that he had crawled through a narrow passage leading into a chamber. In the middle of the cavern was a sunken pool into which steps had been carved. The kahunas chanted and moved their arms, just like Hopis do in certain ceremonies. The head kahuna took Bill to the pool's edge, and asked him to look at the water and tell what he saw.

Bill said he saw ripples that appeared almost as waves on the water's surface. The kahuna asked him to explain their presence.

Bill knew that he saw waves, that the waves were there, but he knew the mountain wasn't moving and that he was higher than sea level. He didn't know *why* there were waves, but he knew the kahuna had asked him an important question. So he answered: "I know there are waves, and I know they are important."

The head kahuna nodded and got undressed, motioning Bill to do so as well. Then they both walked down the stairs into the pool. Soloho's initiation was complete.

The riddle still escaped me, so I asked Bill what the answer was. He laughed and said, "You white people are all the same.

What's the answer? The kahunas didn't know the answer either. Some questions don't have answers. It's enough to know that the question is important."

What we see is not all there is; it's only as much as we can answer now. We will probably never know the whole story.

The kahunas only know that when the pool surface stops rippling, civilization will come to an end. *How* makes no real difference. It's important to recognize the value of questions and to accept the mystery. The willingness not to know it all allows us to be in touch with the more intuitive, creative, unbridled parts of ourselves.

Psychoanalytic theories are so preoccupied with biographical questions of why, how, when, where, that they lose sight of the fact that the answers don't change anything—and sometimes they even interfere.

Years later, I saw Popeye's picture in the newspaper. The caption explained that he was one of the participants to finish in a wheelchair marathon.

We are here for such a brief period of time. We come and go like flickers of a flame. Sometimes we get so serious about what it all means. The important thing is to play the hand you've been dealt.

The Indians take the perspective that death will take care of itself. The past and the future are simply reflections of an everlasting *now*. In this ongoing present reality, we are connected to those who came before and to those who will come after.

We are here to help each other discover our individual uniqueness. This selfhood, once understood, will of itself sustain us and will, in turn, connect us to the larger reality of humans and spiritual experience. In that way, we may all become dancing healers.

Chapter 12

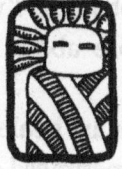

HEALING

When I came to Indian country as a young doctor, I thought I was bringing truth, healing, and knowledge to a backward people. In those first years, I was sometimes met with anger and hostility, other times with indifference. Even the patients who "needed" me the most seemed to shrug their shoulders at my explanations of what could and could not be done to heal them.

I am a better healer now. I have learned that the patient doesn't need a scientist who simply carries out instructions from the laboratory manual. Patients don't want to be cases—they want to be healed. They want to participate in their own wellness or their own death. Patients are the principal agents in their lives, and as much as they want to be well, they want peace and understanding. To find such a healing peace they need to feel that a connection exists between themselves and the healer and between themselves and something larger than self or science.

What patients believe about the doctor's ability to heal may make the difference in their recovery. It certainly makes a difference in their peace of mind.

As I've continued my quest to become a healer, I've learned many steps from many dancers. It is through these steps that I have become a better doctor, a better psychiatrist. As I've learned to share the steps of others I've discovered my own music. I've learned more about being human and about faith.

We are always patients, and sometimes we are healers. We move from being one to being the other. Sometimes I do the work, and sometimes someone else does the work.

Here are some of my own stories. I hope my mentors will smile at my dance. They have taught me the steps.

"Primitive" Indian cultures have used many powerful natural substances as sacraments. Modern culture tends to abuse these same substances: alcohol, tobacco, hallucinogens, herbs.

The special tobacco the Navajo or the Plains tribes smoke in ceremonies is a mixture of herbs and native tobacco that has meaning for its role in ritual. The smoke gives color and smell to one's words. What is said can be sent on the wings of an eagle to touch God's ear. And the smoke can cleanse the body of the clinging dust of ordinary reality. The power of the smoke comes from mixing your breath with that of others, a reminder that we are all on this path together—people, plants, animals, and air.

The smoke is not "funny" tobacco, and the ritual has nothing to do with smoking cigarettes compulsively. Addiction is the opposite of sacrament. Nothing could be less sacred than consuming a substance habitually until it becomes ordinary and no longer has its special power.

Herbs too have a place in the sacrament of healing, as do

singing songs, burning cedar, waving feathers, holding teddy bears, or any other sign of hope.

Joe, a middle-aged Chippewa traditionalist, built a sweat lodge on his wife's reservation (in spite of the community's disapproval) and used it regularly as a way of dealing with a chronic abdominal pain. He worked as a long-distance truck driver until he decided that if he were to cramp while driving, the danger to himself and others would be too great. He quit driving, but he couldn't stand working inside, and he needed to be his own boss. "Just tell me where you want it; I'll get it there" was as much supervision as he tolerated.

Unable to drive his truck, Joe didn't know what else to do. More accurately, he *believed* there was nothing else he could do. He was afraid to explore other paths, in part because he had dropped out of school and he feared that technical training would require more effort than he believed he could expend.

He was referred to me by the internists who told him they had done all they could for his abdominal cramps. He had heard something about me and he knew I wouldn't judge his sweat lodge practices as peculiar.

He told me his story—about a large abusive family, delinquency, running away, and other run-ins. He had returned to the traditional spiritual path during an incarceration. He had been doing well, was working, and was committed to his family until he got sick.

After listening to his story, I did not interpret Joe's concerns about competence, fear, intelligence, or masculinity. Instead, I had him imagine a voyage inside his abdomen to the afflicted spot. In his imagination, he could breathe in a healing, flexible fiberoptic light, carried in an illuminated air bubble, and allow it to course through his body from his lungs through his heart and into his abdomen, right to the place of pain.

And he saw the pain as an ugly, dark, baseball-sized mass that had an irregular margin with a piece reaching out like a finger. He visualized the finger as a dark tunnel with him inside. He could see a light at its end. I told Joe he would be guided through the tunnel by a source of power that would come to him as an animal.

He saw a giant green moth, of a species that had flown near his childhood home. This creature led him to the light.

Afterwards, I told him that a moth is an interesting animal. It starts out life as an animal that crawls, then it changes and gets wings and becomes an animal that flies. Nothing stays the same. You start rolling and then discover you can fly. He also understood that the green moth was his power animal, and he could use it and depend on it to give him strength, because it was his; it was himself. He could fly.

I also gave Joe some herbs for his stomach recommended by an herbalist, an Anglo woman married to a Navajo, who gathers herbs from untouched places in the desert and sells them all over the world.

Finally, I offered to give him some leads about career counseling and vocational testing, which he accepted a short time later. He did get another job, and he found there was another way to move. And finally his pains disappeared.

People always provide keys like the moth; all of us have the keys to our own enlightenment. The therapist uses whatever symbols mean something to that patient. Patients already have the answers to their questions. As the therapist listens to the problem, the patient will also tell the solution.

When you choose to take the journey of enlightenment, you always find guides. And nothing is so big that you do not already have the resources to meet it.

What we see as science, the Indians see as magic. What we see as magic, they see as science. I don't find this a hopeless contradiction. If we can appreciate each other's views, we can see the whole picture more clearly. To heal ourselves or to help heal others we need to reconnect magic and science, our right and left brains.

Mainstream America is a left-brain culture—we believe in rational scientific thought, causality, explanation. The right brain is the home of magic, of intuition, emotion, creativity, faith, the irrational. Great discoveries in science or art are made through the nonrational, nonlinear insights of the right brain. It is the left brain that knows how to speak, but the right brain that remembers the lyrics to songs. You need both sides to dance. You need both sides to remain healthy.

More and more, psychiatry emphasizes the left brain and the biochemical explanations for all behavior, without equal effort to understand the magic and mystering of healing. And it's the healing that matters, not the techniques or the explanations.

The Indian healers' methods are based in faith, but when their methods don't work, they never hesitate to send a suffering person to a hospital or a white doctor. They use whatever works.

Healing is what works.

Flora was a Mexican-Yaqui woman who had been raised in a series of foster homes. She was repeatedly sexually abused and raped in two of her foster homes. Her mother was said to be a witch, and Flora believed her mother could cast spells. She was afraid to go home, even for a short time.

By the time I met Flora, she had some serious psychiatric problems and relied on pills to remain on an even keel. She had also managed to earn a master's degree and was working as a health professional. Flora was articulate; she presented her history undefensively and was capable of listening, so she was an excellent psychotherapy candidate.

Her most significant breakthrough occurred during a Yaqui Easter ceremony. It was the mystical Indian part of her that seemed to hold some power over Flora. She knew the symbology of the Yaquis' Easter rituals and at some level she believed in their power.

Over several weeks during the holy season, members of the Yaqui tribe enact an elaborate ritual that combines elements of their original Indian faith and the Catholic beliefs they learned from missionaries. On the day before Easter, there is a symbolic burning of a cloth-draped wooden statue of Judas. The statue is paraded into the courtyard in front of the community's Catholic church. The figure is surrounded by musicians and revelers wearing human and animals masks and jingling leg rattles. They are the chapayekas, Judas's entourage, and they are rejoicing over his betrayal of Christ.

But soon Judas will be torched, and the forces of goodness will obliterate the evil and the age of salvation will be born. The ritual not only replicates the Christian story; it also gives participants an opportunity to give up some of their old sins, conflicts, fears, or pains in a symbolic way. People tie offerings of hope and relief to the Judas figure.

Flora did not want to participate in the ceremony, because she did not want to confront her mother. So I told her I would take the offering for her. Flora brought me a scarf of hers and as we talked about her life, she used the scarf to wipe her tears.

I went to the Saturday ceremony at the Yaqui village of Guadalupe. At the appropriate time, I tied Flora's tear-stained scarf carrying her painful history and my hope for her relief to the Judas figure. No one stopped or questioned me; no one stops seekers from realizing their hope. As the Judas burned, I felt, in addition to the horror, a sense of hope, even awe, at the power of this setting.

Flora's healing came equally from the burning of her tear-stained past and from my tying it to the Judas. In addition to the negative force of her mother's power, she had an even stronger conviction that she could find relief. Her belief was bolstered by the knowledge that I had taken it all seriously enough to perform the ritual. Flora did much better; she soon left the state, and left much of her painful past behind.

Walking the path together promotes the healing process.

One of my patients was a twenty-year-old Anglo woman, the daughter of a dear friend. Less than six months after her marriage, a large inoperable tumor was discovered in her neck. A cancer of the lymph glands, it extended into her chest. It was responsive to chemo- and radiotherapy, but the chemicals made Tracy sick; even the smells in the oncologist's waiting room made her throw up.

Tracy's husband and family tried to get her to take the treatments, but she felt too weak. She spent her days watching television soap operas, interrupted only for appointments with the radiation therapist. Finally, her mother-in-law prevailed on her at least to talk to someone outside the family, hoping someone would convince Tracy to go for chemotherapy.

But Tracy's agenda was different. She didn't want the chemotherapy now. She was skeletal, jaundiced, weak, and she wanted to know what I believed. Did I believe, as she did, that this would pass and then she would be okay?

I talk about these things now—not just what the patient believes, but also what I believe, how I understand the mysterious.

Tracy talked about childhood friends and the ocean and her wedding picture and her dog. During these days, Tracy imagined this peaceful scene: she saw herself as a little girl in a meadow of flowers and clover, with protective trees. She could visualize a rickety bridge leading over a creek. The other side was not clear, but she could cross the bridge, and if she felt frightened she could hold onto supports around her. The rail was her husband's hand, and her grandmother's, and her dog was beside her on the way.

I said that each life is a series of bridges. We cross new ones as we move from one life phase to another. Sometimes the bridges reach over chasms of pain, of fear, or of sadness. And the only way to make it across is to be supported by something that reminds you that you are not alone.

In her peaceful meadow, Tracy once rode on the back of a giant eagle and soared above the bridge to look at the dark side. It was less forbidding than she had feared. When the great bird landed she saw herself dismounting into the hands of loved ones.

I shared my beliefs and values with Tracy. I talked about my own pain and my own connections. I sang to her in Hebrew and English a song of the Hasidic master, Reb Nachman of Bratislav. He taught that the unknown is an adventure, and the way to make it through was not to fear.

> The whole world is just a narrow bridge.
> Just a narrow bridge, and
> Above all, above all,
> Is not to fear,
> Not to fear, at all.

Eight weeks after I first saw Tracy she died. She had kept the tape of my song and stories at her bedside. She played it twice a day to help her rest. I feel as good about giving her this as I would as if I had been able to persuade her to go for chemotherapy.

My old Jewish connections keep coming back to me. Every time I think I've got my identity clear, something happens to remind me of those connections. I had been raised in a conservative, if not absolutely observant, Jewish home. As a young man I rejected this part of my past because it didn't have all the answers. In the radicalism of the 1960s, many of us dismissed any and all traditions in an attempt to free ourselves from hypocrisy—we threw the baby out with the bath.

In Santa Fe, I tried to raise my children with the consciousness of universalists, as members of the tribe of humankind. They would learn to believe in the unity of humankind, not to follow restrictive practices of one tribe.

Then one day the children decided they wanted to go to church with their friends in this very Catholic town. I suddenly rediscovered the force of my attachment to the old connection. This happened at the same time that I was learning another dance from the Pueblos and the power of their connections. The reality hit me: my children didn't know what they were. They didn't really know what it meant to be a Jew. I discovered that it mattered to me what they were, what I was. It was a connection of truth and one of credibility. This is my tribe. So we began going to the synagogue again. In the absence of our circuit-riding rabbi, I even filled in for him a few times.

All tribes, all religions, are sustained by similar myths — births, rebirths, faith in miracles. These stories, these connections to our way, are the predicates on which all morality is based. They are what sustains us as good people in the hard times. I came to realize that you have to know who you are before you can be a universalist; it's what makes us each unique that lets us appreciate the universalities among us. If you can realize that your heritage is part of what makes you special, then you can realize that others are special too.

In time, however, I found organized Jewish worship a difficult place to feel the spirit. The synagogue was the least spiritual place I knew. On the holiest days, great throngs and multiple distractions made it hard to be serious about prayer. It was in the tipi or the sweat lodge that I was best able to see the face of Abraham, to huddle with Jacob in the desert, to feel the presence of a spirit in the coals of a fire.

Lately a small group of friends and I have spent these holy days creating our own liturgy. We prepare ourselves for the penance of the Days of Awe in our own sweat lodge. It is built with the traditional frame of twelve willow branches; I see them as the tribes of Israel.

In the circle, we pass sacred objects and each participant talks. We recall our desert ancestry and our connections to the Earth. We sing the old melodies, we burn cedar, we recreate in the small group a circle of faith, a place of prayer. Prayer is an expression of the heart that goes directly to the tongue without first being short-circuited by the brain.

Every day, in many ways, in unexpected places, you can hear a new tune and learn another step in your dance.

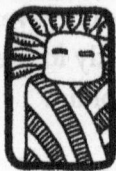

Chapter 13

THE SUN DANCE

I first heard about Brave Buffalo from Basil, my Phoenix Indian High School friend who, after graduation, became involved in the American Indian Movement. After participating in marches and military confrontations for a time, he found himself on the Indian spiritual path—the "Red Road." He became involved with a traditional Indian spiritual community in Portland, Oregon, called Anpo, the Lakota Sioux word for "dawn."

Anpo is a realization of the vision of Brave Buffalo, a Brule Sioux. The community conducts Indian-sensitive teaching programs for the Portland public schools; it sponsors museum exhibitions, dances, and craft fairs. Brave Buffalo has lectured about traditional Indian beliefs all over America and Europe. He has a fifth-grade education, but he has much to say.

Once a year, in July (the Moon of Making Fat), Brave Buffalo sponsors a Sun Dance. He had a dream telling him to recreate the sacred hoop of the Sun Dance, the most sacred ceremony of the Plains tribes, which include the Sioux.

If you have a vision and believe in its validity, you have to do what it commands. You have to share it with others;

otherwise it's like a gift that remains forever unopened.

For the last four years, Anpo has sponsored a Sun Dance on grounds in the Mt. Hood National Forest. The Forest Service closes the area to other users during the four days of the ceremony.

The participants in the Sun Dance believe that if Indian people come together again in this sacred circle, civilization will endure. If they fulfill this commitment made by their ancestors to Wakan Tanka, the Great Spirit, then the earth will survive.

The dancers dance not for themselves alone, but for their families, their tribes, and for all of humankind. As a gesture of surrender to the Creator, warriors pierce their flesh with sticks. They believe their flesh is the only thing they can offer to the Creator that is truly their own.

Black Elk, the Sioux visionary and Keeper of the Sacred Pipe, spoke of the Sun Dance in this way:

> We hold it during the Moon of Making Fat, because this is the time when the sun is at its highest and the growing power of the world is strongest. We select the sacred tree. The people come to it singing, with flowers all over them. A brave warrior strikes the living tree, counting coup on it [from the practice in warfare of hitting a fallen enemy with a stick, which then counted him as a casualty], because the spirit of the sun loves everything that bears fruit. Then maidens chop it down. We carry it home, stopping four times, once for each season and direction, to give thanks for this gift of life. Then the sacred tree is set down at a place in the center. We plant it in the earth; we make a vow to the Great Spirit, Wakan Tanka.
>
> This tree is the center of the living universe. It holds the power of the world. It is the centerpiece of the four

directions. The East brings peace and light; the South, warmth; the West brings rain; and the North, strength and endurance.

The sky is the great circle that surrounds us. The earth is the circle that supports us. The sun comes and goes in a great circle just like our lives.

Everything in life is a great circle; the tipis are round like the nests of birds—they hold the children who are the guardians of our immortality. And we are, in turn, embraced by the Earth Mother who in her roundness provides us with the fruitfulness of life.

On the morning before the Sun Dance, nursing mothers bring their little ones to be blessed at the base of the tree of life, here at the center of the universe. Grow up and be brave; make your people proud.

Holy men will pierce their ears. The dancers paint their bodies; they lay beneath the tree and the holy men cut places in their backs or chest so they can fulfill their oaths. Each man thus fastened to the tree gets up and dances until his flesh tears loose.

This is the dancers' pledge: I give you this piece of my spirit, give me the peace of your presence. I touch your presence on this Mother Earth; treat me with kindness and give my people life.

By the beginning of the twentieth century, the Sun Dance had been outlawed as a barbaric ritual. The offering of living flesh as a sacrifice was deemed a degenerate and primitive practice. The Sioux later petitioned the courts, saying that fulfilling this sacred obligation was necessary to ensure their lives, indeed the lives of everyone on earth. Eventually, the government relented and permitted the Sun Dance—but without piercing. With the passage of the Native American Religious Freedoms Act in 1978 public piercing was again allowed.

When I attended the Sun Dance, I thought I'd be one of the few non-Indians. It turns out there were Germans, French, Japanese, Rastafarians, Christians, Jews, Mormons, and Buddhists. Mostly, there were Indian people from tribes all over the hemisphere — hundreds of people, all together for this seeking of the spirit.

The sacred grounds look like an Edward Curtis photograph of nineteenth-century Indian life. A semicircle of tipis surrounds the Sacred Hoop. At the center, inside a branch-covered arbor, stands the Sun Dance pole; it's about fifty feet high and draped with scarves of red, white, yellow, and black, the colors of the four directions.

Wrapped around the trunk are ropes, one for each dancer who has tied his own spiritual lifeline to the tree. Once he ties the rope, it has to be used, otherwise his spirit can't be released. If a dancer becomes sick or for some other reason can't be pierced, someone else must complete the ritual for him. At the very top of the tree an eagle feather and two leather figurines, one, a man, the other a buffalo, both danced in the breeze.

Surrounding the pole, at a radius of maybe fifty feet, is a covered arbor under which all the supporters stand, except at the open east end of the circle. Dawn's first ray must strike the sacred tree unobstructed.

At the western edge of the arbor is a covered ramada where the dancers rest between dance rounds. Behind it is an enclosed compound with three tipis and sweat lodges. The dancers stay in the compound without eating or drinking for four days.

They enter the sweat lodges twice daily. Even after four days, they still sweat. I don't know how they do it with no fluid intake. In medical school, I was taught that the body could not survive without water after three days because the kidneys start to shut down.

After days of prayer and preparation, the Sun Dance begins at dawn. Everyone is called to the arbor by a raucous symphony of eagle-bone whistles. Each dancer wears a whistle around his neck and blows it while moving. I hear the cry in my sleeping bag and feel like a target in Alfred Hitchcock's movie *The Birds*.

The first to enter the circle is a Horned Buffalo Dancer; he carries a "smudge pot," a number-10 can filled with burning sage; he brushes the smoke into the arbor with an eagle feather to sanctify the place and its occupants. All present are now in the center of all things. This cleansing ritual separates us from every influence outside the circle: from the worries, pain, antagonisms, and ordinary fears of daily life, from all except the feeling of the spirit within the hoop.

Pregnant women are welcomed under the arbor because this place is a good influence on unborn children, but menstruating women are not allowed into the circle. They are not excluded in shame, but in recognition of their special power and influence at this time.

At the south side of the circle is the great drum. Its rhythms behind the chanted melodies captivate us with their vibrations. My feet move; my body sways. The songs says, "Wakan Tanka—Great Spirit—here we are at the center; we have only you in our minds."

Following the Buffalo Dancer comes a woman cradling the sacred pipe. She represents the White Buffalo Calf Woman who originally brought the sacred pipe to the people and instructed them in its use.

Into the red pipestone bowl is carved a figure of the sacred buffalo, the bringer of all goodness, which fed, clothed, housed, and sustained the people. Beneath the bowl is an eagle feather for the sacred brother whose wings touch the ear of the Creator, Wakan Tanka, the bringer of light. Tied to the pipe's shaft are sage and sweet grass, a reminder that if the people bind themselves to the Spirit in this sacred way, then they will multiply and the earth endure.

The Lakota smoke the pipe whenever they conduct sacred business. The pipe ceremony prepares any setting for truth. Like the smoke smudging, it separates the ordinary from the extraordinary, the profane from the sacred. When you share the smoke, the breath of your life spirit, with others in the spirit of truth, something good will happen. They say the pipe has the power of peace, of healing, of life.

Following the Buffalo Calf Woman come the warriors. Each wears a Sun Dance skirt from waist to ankles. Each enters the hoop, cradling his own pipe in his forearm. Then come the women; they too carry their own pipes. Inside the hoop, the sixty dancers stop at each of the four directions. Then they enter the covered resting place, placing their pipes against a forked stick altar before entering.

After each dance round, six or seven dancers pick up their pipes in an exchange ceremony. On the south side, they give it to someone picked from among the supporters, who then invites others to share it. By day's end, every pipe will have been exchanged and smoked by hundreds of people.

During most rounds, some dancers are pierced. When it is a dancer's turn, he lies on a buffalo-hide rug at the base of the sacred tree, while holy men make two parallel incisions to lift a finger-width strip of skin on each side of his chest or his back with a surgical scalpel. A round, sharpened piece of wood is thrust under the skin. No one cries out during the piercing.

The peg is fastened to the dancer's rope which is tied to the Sun Dance pole. Each dancer walks backwards as far as his rope allows and, leaning away from the pole, he dances until the skin breaks. That moment is one of liberation. The dancer, in triumph, circles the hoop joyfully. Some whose backs are pierced drag buffalo skulls behind them around the perimeter of the circle until the skin breaks. The moment of release is one of ecstasy.

I do not have difficulty with the ordeal. The Sacred Pole is a Tree of Life, as the Torah of the Jews is "a tree of life to those who hold fast to it," says the Talmud. Jews reminds themselves of this gift every morning at dawn. They bind leather straps on their arms and heads as a commitment that their hearts and minds must stay connected to this tree of life if they as a people are to survive. Indeed, the healing of the earth depends upon their doing this. The Lakotas' Sun Dance is remarkably similar in purpose and symbol.

During the evenings and early morning hours of the Sun Dance, everyone in the camp can participate in sweat ceremonies. The sweat lodges go long into the night, as long as there are people waiting. Like the Sun Dance and the pipe, they are sacred ceremonies. Inside the sweat lodge, the pipe is passed to each participant. Everyone holds it, smokes it, and gets a turn to speak.

At my turn, I sing a song in Hebrew and find myself joined by another voice! Here, in the middle of the eastern Oregon forest, at a sacred Indian ceremony, I am singing in Hebrew and with another member of my tribe! The power of this moment fills me with a sense of the spirit in this place. In the blackness, I am moved to tears. I am unashamed because I cannot be seen, but I feel naked before the spirit.

On the afternoon of the third day, Brave Buffalo calls me into the circle to receive a pipe in the exchange from one of the warriors. It is an honor to be called forth. As the young warrior approaches me with his pipe, he stops and whispers to the leader that he doesn't want to exchange it with me. I don't know whether he has picked someone else, or if he dislikes me or maybe white people in general. But I feel that he ought to be able to choose anyone he wants to support him during this ordeal. I am asked to step back and somebody else comes forward.

Brave Buffalo later tells me that what happened really isn't the way. You don't refuse to exchange your pipe if someone has been selected to come forward to receive it; it is in the exchange that one actually understands the meaning of the Sun Dance. When people share that pipe they fulfill the prophetic message of the coming together of all the peoples and colors of the four directions in a harmony of Spirit to perpetuate the earth and everything that lives on it.

I told myself I was not hurt by the warrior's rejection, but I was.

The next day I am called forward again. I would have been happy to stay back; I didn't want to be refused again. But if you're picked, you are expected to participate even if you don't feel ready to; someone else must feel you are and that's why you were picked. That degree of trust encourages one to get out of old conditioning and take a chance at spontaneity.

I step forward and, as only happens in the movies, I find myself opposite the same dancer who refused me the day before. This time he offers me his pipe. I appreciate what his choosing to approach me again says about him.

We stand not more than two feet apart and look at each other, but we don't speak. Four times we reach out to each other, and on the last time he gives me his sacred pipe. I smoke the pipe with others and tell them how pleased I am to have stepped forward and confronted my fear of rejection (my ego, my narcissism). When I return his pipe to him, we look at each other again, still silent.

That night I dream about my daughter and her boyfriend, a very nice guy, but not a member of my tribe. Because he didn't know my songs and dances, and I think he doesn't care, I've judged him badly. In my dream I see the two of them in some imminent danger. I rush to warn them of a disaster, but they can't seem to hear me. I am stopped by an invisible plastic shield that insulates them. I scream and bang on it, but they do not hear me. I am feeling more desperation and wake up with a start, sweating, my heart pounding.

In the predawn light I understand what I came to the Sun Dance to learn. That dancer judged me as unacceptable, for whatever reason. But he chose to come back to me. I judged the boyfriend, but I never came back to him, and now I was about to lose my daughter.

When the Sun Dance ends, the dancers emerge from the circle for the first time since they entered four days earlier. They greet the rest of us who are lined up outside. I shake hands and hold the dancer with whom I exchanged the pipe. Still, we don't speak.

That night at the celebration, I tell Brave Buffalo about my dream. I wonder aloud whether to seek out the dancer to share my insight and thank him. Brave Buffalo asks, "Why?

You only understand it as you understand it. How you see it is just the way it is for you. For him too it is as it is. The hope is that we try to see it in as many ways and as many times as we can."

So this is how I see it for now:

Once I was comfortable only with speaking words; I have since learned to sing, to pray, to touch. I reveal and I listen; I sometimes light candles and cedar. Whenever I used only one dimension in the healing process, I minimized my potential healing power. I had to feel my power to know it, and now I can't imagine it differently. There is a world beyond our own awareness.

The Sioux, the Cheyenne, the Assiniboin, the Blackfeet, and the Mandan were defeated by war and disease. The great buffalo were rendered nearly extinct; the people of the Plains were deprived of a way of life, but not of their spirit.

When Black Elk was an old man, he asked to be taken back to the Sacred Mountain where he first saw his vision. There he spoke to the Great Spirit, Wakan Tanka.

> Grandfather, with tears, I say to you that our nation's hoop is broken and scattered. This is not the center any longer. The sacred tree does not bloom here. Where you took me when I was young and taught me, here I stand now, as an old man, in sorrow and feeble voice. The tree is withered. If some little root still lives, may it leaf and bloom and fill with singing birds. May it bloom not for myself but for my people that they may once more go back to the sacred hoop and find the good Red Road, the Shielding Tree.

It is a tree of life to those who hold fast to it. Everyone needs a tree.

Kallah

After the Sun Dance sweat lodge ceremony, as we all mingled outside, a man approached me and thanked me for my song. He said he had thought about singing in Hebrew but wondered whether it was appropriate.

I repeated, as I had heard it, that as long as you had a language in which you prayed and a song that carried its message, it was always appropriate. At least you and the Creator understand the words, and the others will appreciate your efforts.

I thanked him too. In all my experience in Indian country, I told him, this was the first time anybody had ever joined me in singing in my own language. How moved I felt, indeed how awed, to be in this isolated, spiritual place and to find there a member of my tribe.

Aryeh turned out to be a rabbi. He came to the Sun Dance because here he could feel the spirit. He held feathers as he danced, and he brought his prayer shawl and phylacteries—those leather straps of devotion—to greet the morning sun.

Aryeh received his ordination from a New Age Hasidic rabbi, Reb Zalman Schacter. Reb Zalman was trained by the Lubavitch Hasidim in Brooklyn. In the fomenting 1960s he found a ready audience of young Jews who responded to his mystical worldview.

Reb Zalman at first went to Canada and later became a professor of Jewish Mysticism at Temple University and a teacher at the Reconstructionist Rabbinical College in Philadelphia. He is also "Rebbe in Residence" and founder of B'nai Or, the Followers of Light, a traditionally oriented Jewish community organized around the belief that all learning takes place within the context of a spiritual life and that one can expand old religious paradigms to find new ways to experience awe. Reb Zalman also ordains rabbis, which is a little bit controversial in the organized hierarchy of official learning.

Aryeh asked me to join him in morning prayers the following day. It had been a long time since I had greeted the sun in the company of another Jew. I joined him in my prayer shawl, the same one I wear in the tipi. Aryeh wore a prayer shawl of many colors such as I had never seen before.

In the morning, as we sang in Hebrew, Ivdu HaShem b'simcha, "Worship God with Joy," I heard in the distance the Sun Dancers entering the sacred circle and blowing their eagle-bone whistles. It is the first time I can remember greeting the dawn with tears.

Here in Indian country my heart again opened to an appreciation of the mystery. For a long time this part of me had cried to be filled, but I did not want to acknowledge this need. Here, in the unassuming simplicity of the ceremonies, I felt a connection to a sense of the infinite and an appreciation of the spirit in the small things I had too long taken for granted.

My wife is not moved in the ways I am at Indian spiritual gatherings. She yearned to touch that part of herself in a Jewish environment and was frightened by my growing distance from it.

After our morning service, I asked Aryeh about the multicolored prayer shawl. He told me it was the result of a Reb Zalman vision, a dream about the biblical account of how God wrapped himself in a "cloak of light" before creating the universe. Zalman saw the shawl as having all the colors of the rainbow; he says he no longer sees things as just black or white.

As soon as I got home, I sent away to find out more about B'nai Or.

The following year, almost at the exact time of the previous year's Sun Dance, B'nai Or sponsored a Kallah or spiritual retreat. It would include a "vision quest." A rabbi, inspired by a Lakota spiritual leader with whom he studied, had translated an Indian worldview into a Jewish liturgical experience. We would meet as a tribe the evening before our quest and prepare ourselves to respond to God's challenge to Abraham and Sarah to reach beyond themselves in order to find their deepest selves. It was an offer I could not refuse, and it seemed made to order as a way for my wife, Elaine, and me to reexperience a Jewish spiritual rootedness.

We participated in workshops on future visioning and mask-making, dancing and praying from the inside. The vision quest was held on the Sabbath eve.

The evening before, sixty of us meet as a group. The Rebbe lights sage and passes it around in an abalone shell.

He talks about questing from a Jewish mystical perspective: how both concepts emphasize solitude, you go alone to seek enlightenment; how both require ritual cleansing and the use of objects and special garments to protect oneself from evil influences. Both acknowledge spirit messages and messengers. Both encourage altered states of consciousness through deprivation, fasting, and prayer, and in both there is the hope of receiving guidance through the spirit.

We sing the ancient chants, and each of us picks a card on which is written one word that is to serve as a meditation focus in tomorrow's silence. Mine says "knowingness."

Before dawn the following morning, we gather in an oak grove to recite the morning prayers. The Rebbe has picked selections from the liturgy that I had never heard: prayers about guardian spirits, animals, the earth, and the four directions.

The morning is shrouded in a misty fog. With the first light, some stand and wrap the leather straps of devotion to their arms and heads. In the distance, thunder rumbles while we chant, "The Earth, the Water, the Fire, the Air, Return Return Return." I feel again the tears at dawn.

The morning service breaks; it is now the time of silence and solitude. I wander silently, my prayer shawl draped on my shoulders. I stroll through a Catholic college campus with religious statuary everywhere and smile to think how Mother Cabrini would appreciate the scene. I smell a flower, and for a long, long time watch an inchworm slowly cross a leaf; it is a modern dancer.

Sitting on a playground swing, I think psychotherapy is a vision quest with the psychiatrist as guide to help facilitate the experience.

I walk up a hill and come upon the Rebbe in a tree. He is *in* the tree—not on a branch but sitting inside a cavelike hollow in its trunk. He sits totally enveloped by his prayer shawl.

"The Rebbe in a tree." The music of it, the clarity: "the Rebbe is in a tree." In every tree, a Rebbe, in every tree and in every thing. There is a spirit in all things.

When I come to the next tree, I wrap my arms around it. I feel it; I feel its aliveness; it hums. A bug crawls out of the tree, right under my nose, and I can feel its steps—it dances. I have never looked at a bug so closely.

Continuing my walk, I am caught by surprise again: here in the middle of Pennsylvania, right in the middle of an amphitheater, I have come upon a tipi. I discovered that I have wandered onto the grounds of a military academy that uses the tipi for some ceremonial occasion.

Today it's just standing there empty. I go inside and take out the cedar I brought with me knowing there would come a time to use it. I fill the tipi with its fragrance. A soft rain against the tipi's outside sounds like music on a canvas drum. I enshroud myself with my prayer shawl.

I am the Rebbe in this tree. Everyone of us a Rebbe. We are the language of the creative source and with all things we are as kin. Again I feel tears of unexplainable joy.

I remember my word: "knowingness." I don't "know" how I found this place but I know I want to experience it again. This is what I want to be, to accept things as I experience them and accept that there are things I will never "know."

This openness makes life's journey not only tolerable but allows us, again and again, to experience awe. Awe: that moment of insight into meaning other than ourselves, meaning in the small things that help us recognize the presence of the infinite.

A couple of weeks after the Kallah, I attended the Big Mountain Sun Dance. Sitting under the covered arbor day after day was a paralyzed woman in a wheelchair. She had use only of her fingers, just enough to move an electrical switch to control the movement of her chair. To get to the arbor, she had to be pushed along a rugged path. Once she arrived, she stayed all day.

On the afternoon of the third day, a warrior (himself crippled with a shriveled leg), was struggling to drag the skulls attached to the wooden pins in the flesh of his back. Already weak, he had twice circled the hoop. Friends and relatives entered the circle to stand behind him. Fanning him with feathers, they whispered encouragement.

In my heart, I wanted to step inside and be part of this group, but my feet would not move. (I don't know this man. What will others think?) My heart speaks, but my feet have a mind of their own.

The woman in the wheelchair asked somebody to push her into the circle. As a young man pushed her among those who followed the struggling Sun Dancer, she came to a complete stop directly in front of me—the wheels of the chair were sunk in six inches of sand. Had she stopped a foot in front of me or behind me I would have been spared the need to decide to step forward. My feet carried me, and while the other man pulled, I pushed her. Together we moved around the circle.

Here was a woman who was totally immobilized but whose heart, mind, and body followed the harmony of her truth. She knew she wanted to step in, so she did it. Yet I, who can move, needed her direct invitation to connect with my truth.

Sometimes it is the crippled who help us walk and the blind who help us see. What do I know? I know that had she not stopped directly in front of me, I would not have moved.

She stopped to help me move. In this small thing I sense the awesome presence of the mysterious.

Chapter 14

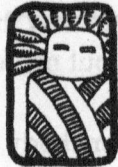

BEAR BUTTE

In the fall of 1985 I addressed a conference of Indian hospital program directors on the subject of "Indian Perspectives on Healing." The conference was held in Rapid City, South Dakota, a place I had wanted to visit for a long time.

The Black Hills of South Dakota and Bear Butte are most sacred places for the Sioux, the Cheyenne, and all the tribes of the Plains. It was to this sacred mountain called Bear Butte that Red Cloud came for help and guidance before the so-called Red Cloud Wars. This is the place of Crazy Horse, Sitting Bull, and Black Elk; and it is here that the Cheyenne received the four sacred arrows that still sustain the spiritual life of their people.

Here also friends whom I call relatives have come on their own vision quests, to spend up to four days and nights on the peak seeking enlightenment. Bear Butte is a place of spiritual reflection, a place to seek direction, to look at what purpose you serve—a place of decision.

I wanted to experience this sacred place, but I did not anticipate that this visit would add this closing chapter to my years in Indian country, a step in my seeking to become a healer, in my own vision quest.

Before my trip to Bear Butte I visited the Sioux Indian Museum in downtown "Rapid." The museum was offering items for sale as part of a building fund drive. On one table I spotted a seventy-five-year-old elaborately beaded and quilled Sioux tobacco pouch. I could not resist. With the pouch came a small pipe. I also bought rattle used by the Yuwipi medicine men in the healing ceremonies of the Sioux.

As I drove toward Bear Butte, I thought, why not carry the sacred instruments to the peak? It was a unique chance to rededicate them to the purpose for which they were intended. I wanted to accept them in a good way, to say that I would keep them and use them the best way I knew how, and to cleanse them and me from whatever negative influences might interfere with such a recommitment. I felt good about the decision as I drove toward Bear Butte.

Bear Butte is a sacred place, and it's also a state park open to everyone. It has a ranger station, a small museum, marked trails, and lookout platforms; at its base live a small herd of buffalo. The butte rises like a volcanic marble two thousand feet above the flat plains. It has served as a landmark to pioneers and prospectors, to the cavalry and Custer.

On this drizzly day with clouds hanging low in the sky not many people were at the park. The ranger station was closed. I parked in the lot at the trail base, took a backpack from the trunk of my car, and laid the pipe and pouch on top of it. As I locked the car a young woman approached me.

Seeing the instruments she asked if I was going to load my pipe and pray on the sacred peak. I said I was going to dedicate my instruments there. Tearfully she told me that her grandmother had died the previous day. She and her relatives had come today to pray for her journey. Would I remember her in my prayers? she asked. I felt honored to do so.

She spoke of her grandmother, and I listened. It felt good to communicate this way. There were no questions about pedigree, blood, or tribe, just a shared appreciation of the power of the instruments and the sacramental quality of the place.

I packed the things and jauntily started walking toward the sweat lodges at the volcano's base. Feeling cheerful, happy with my purchase, glad to be in this place, gratified by the stranger's confidence, I sauntered up the path. As I approached the grounds, I was stopped cold by a rattling sound. Eighteen inches in front of me a rattlesnake was coiled into striking position, its head flattened and rattle humming. I moved back gingerly. I had never been so close to a rattler in the wild. I started talking to it.

"Be cool. I know you were here first, this is your place. I'm moving back. Be cool." Then, with a flush of societal embarrassment, I looked around to see if anyone was watching me talk to a snake.

Indians have a special thing about snakes. They see them as messengers that move like lightning. Pay attention when these animal brothers move, their entire beings are in contact with the Earth; they can hear the heartbeat of the Earth Mother with their whole body. We are in contact with it only with our feet.

It is the animals who tell us of forthcoming earthquakes, not machines or people. Snakes carry a message about the place where we live: if you don't treat this place carefully, if you march too merrily, if you don't take this place and your purpose on it seriously, something bad will happen. I got the message: don't step lightly. Be serious about what you're here for, what you are about to do, how others have come here before you. This is a sacred place. Don't get captivated by your ego.

I appreciated the reminder; I needed it. I approached the sweat lodge grounds with a wholly different kind of bounce.

Two sweat-lodge frames of willow had been erected. All around them trees were covered with ribbons, scarves, tobacco-filled cloth pouches in the colors of the four directions; even the bushes had the red, yellow, white, and black ties on their branches. Feathers tied to prayer sticks were implanted in front of the lodge frames. The colors fluttered everywhere. You could feel them, like living ornaments blowing wishes.

I shivered with the power of the place and felt the presence of a hundred years of initiates who had come here to prepare for the quest. I touched the pipe rack, the altar, the prayer stick, then tied my own offerings. I continued climbing the path and watched the Great Plains stretch out below. I could see circling wagons and hear screaming warriors. I could see the earth black with buffalo and feel it move with their stampeding. The place was filled with the energy of imagination.

On the hike up the well-traveled trail of Bear Butte I could see colored cloth prayer offerings everywhere, some with tiny items tied in them. In some trees stones are embedded, placed there years before by the faithful.

And paths branching from the main trail are blocked by signs that say: "Indians Praying: Do Not Disturb." How wonderful! We need such signs in every state park, in every forest, and on every waterway. It changes your whole way of looking at a place if you know people are praying there, that the Earth is the cathedral. It says more about why we should respect the Earth than "Don't Step on the Grass," "Keep Out," or "Do Not Litter."

Indians Praying. Do Not Disturb.

At the peak, a marker on a tree cautions hikers not to continue. These are the vision quest grounds.

I feel my hands tingling. The trees are covered with prayer scarves. On both sides of the slopes, as far as my eye can see, rectangles of at least four square feet are formed by strings connected to four trees. The strings are dotted with tiny cloth bundles filled with tobacco and flesh offerings.

During the quest one of these enclosures becomes the center of all things. Here the vision quester sits for days, without eating. A doorway is created by placing two pieces of sage over one of the strings; the quester can enter and exit the space through this "door"; When he or she is inside, the sage is removed.

Here a quester might touch the spark of light that we call insight.

How we need such sacramental places. They don't have to be on a mountaintop or in a temple. Each of us can find this place on our own path, a place that speaks to us in a special way. We make it sacred by separating it from the ordinary world by physical markings or by our attitude. We need to find and recognize the sacred places on our path, to go back to them for sustenance, for centering.

I find an enclosed rectangle nestled into the western slope. I will stay for a while. I leave my pack outside, collect two forked sticks and a cross bar. In the sacred place I make a pipe rack and rest my instruments on it. I light some cedar I brought from Arizona.

I pray. Prayer is whenever you allow your tongue and lips to move synchronously with your heart without first processing your feelings through your head.

The smoke's fragrance bathes me; it separates this place from the ordinary. It removes the lampshades that keep me from appreciating my own light.

I pray about friends, family, ancestors, animals, and the dead grandmother. I pray about my future. In the drizzle, I offer the pipe. My life breath is illuminated in smoke; it seems to make the raindrops stop in midair.

As I sit I wonder how I got here. By what path did I come to this point in my life, in my work?

I think, on the mountain, that in my work as a psychiatrist I am another guide for people seeking vision. I am a guide who helps people process life's experience and find the message within about who we are, what our purposes are, what our paths are. What I do is just another ritualized vision quest. My patients invest my workplace and my ceremony with power; if they believe in my language, in what I know, then they can receive what I have to say to them.

Society has endowed psychiatry with the mantle of legitimacy as the best way to help us make sense of our history. But there are so many ways that can allow us a glimpse into meaning. The important thing is to seek a vision on your path and with someone you trust, someone who speaks your language, who appreciates your dance.

If you choose to make the journey, you will always find guides.

On my way down from the top of Bear Butte I picked up some stones to put in my medicine bundle. I would share and thereby remember some of the healing of this place.

Weeks later I again saw the snake – in a dream. Coiled and rattling, it now spoke to me, but I couldn't hear it. I saw the tongue darting but I couldn't hear the words.

Again the snake. It is these seemingly small events that make up the legends of our lives.

I understand now. It is not what the snake says that is important, but what the snake is. It is my power animal, my reminder. I hear it saying, "You are the messenger. Tell the story before the earth quakes."

So this is the story. I've shared the steps that I learned the best way I know how. I hope they help you to hear your music.

To receive information about Dr. Hammerschlag's workshops, retreats, and lectures, or to order his tapes, please contact him at the following address:

3104 East Camelback Road, #614
Phoenix, Arizona 85016
Phone: (602) 468-1141
Fax: (602) 954-8560